STEPPING STONES

TO YOUR

DREAM ACHIEVEMENT

I0136118

CATHERINE
RAWLING

First published in Australia by Aurora House

This edition published 2025
Copyright © Catherine Rawling 2025

Typesetting and e-book design: Amit Dey (amitdey2528@gmail.com)
Cover design: Donika Mishineva (www.artofdonika.com)

The right of Catherine Rawling to be identified as Author of the Work
has been asserted in accordance with the Copyright, Designs and
Patents Act 1988.

ISBN number: 978-1-923298-31-6 (paperback)

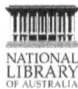

A catalogue record for this
book is available from the
NATIONAL LIBRARY OF AUSTRALIA
National Library of Australia

DEDICATION

This book is dedicated to all those who have a dream but are struggling to see that dream realised. May this book help to shine a light on your pathway towards great success and inspirational living.

CONTENTS

The sacred wisdom and life guidance you are searching for
is hidden in the springtime breeze that flows across the calm
ocean, in the sounds of the birds welcoming in the new day.

When you rest in this moment and connect to nature,
you connect to your heart centre
and this is where you will find the answers
you have been searching for.

INTRODUCTION

A great dream for the future is what will help you get out of bed in the morning, inspired and eager to start the day. A great dream will also help reveal what the next step is. And if you work each day towards your dream achievement, you'll begin to create a beautiful life.

My journey towards living the life of my dreams began when I was eighteen and there was a knock on the door. Someone was announcing the opening of a local karate class in our area. Despite my parents' initial reservations—stemming from misconceptions about karate's ties to religion—I decided to join the class and pursue something I came to be passionate about. I learned the power of focus, discipline and strength in body and mind. Around the same time, I developed a keen interest in self-development. This drive stayed with me through life's highs and lows, fuelling a hunger to continually learn, grow and refine my skill set on a daily basis.

Two years into my karate training, I attended a wellness fair. At one of the stalls, there was a tai chi master who spoke about the profound benefits of tai chi and qigong. Intrigued, I began learning tai chi once a week and practised the new techniques daily alongside my karate.

The combination of the soft, flowing skills of tai chi and the dynamic, powerful techniques of karate created a balanced and rewarding practice. This enhanced my abilities, which led to success in tournaments. I began filling the house with trophies.

At twenty-one, I represented Australia in the World Karate Championships held in Canada and won first place in the performance of a second dan kata. I took home a six-foot trophy and appeared in the local paper with the headline *Karate kid took on the world, and she won.*

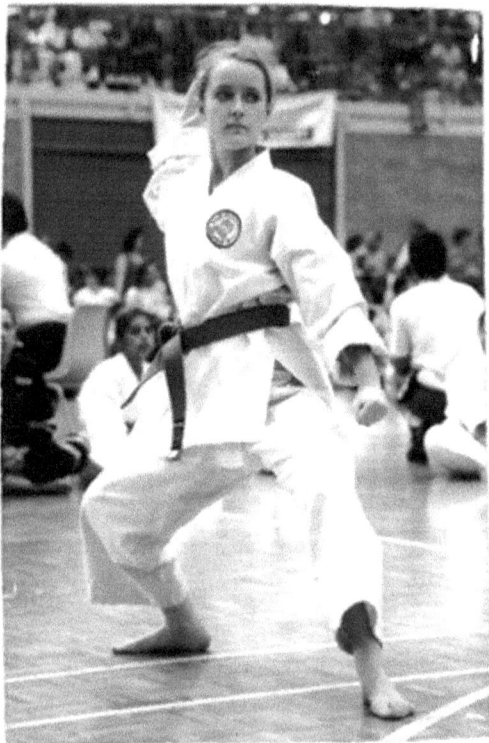

All was going well, but, in my thirties, my desire to own a home and take on a mortgage required full-time work. Before long, I found myself in an unfulfilling administration job and with a house filled with clutter. At that time, I was only focused on survival—paying the bills and trying to keep the house tidy. Then came a series of wake-up calls that made me realise it was time to change and improve my way of living.

The first arrived when I decided to clear the clutter from my house. While sorting through the garage, I stumbled upon a dusty folder containing dreams and goals I had written down a decade earlier—visions of being in a career dedicated to helping others live their dreams.

The second not-so-subtle wake-up call came one night at 10pm. Just as I was drifting off to sleep, a car crashed through my front window. An elderly neighbour was learning to drive, and she had accidentally placed her foot on the accelerator instead of the brake and lost control of the car. I believe this was a literal sign from the universe to wake up, to be more aware and to question whether the path I was travelling on was the right one. It was time for a change. It was time for me to do and be what I was meant to in life.

The third wake-up call arrived when my second-hand car, which I had purchased about six months earlier, broke down on a highway. There I was, sitting on the side of the road with smoke emitting from the engine. It had blown a gasket and was completely unrepairable. This was not the first time that car had broken down. In the months and weeks prior, it had broken down many times, causing much inconvenience. This wake-up call made me question: Why am I in this situation?

How should I improve my life and my finances so something like this does not happen again?

I completed the process of decluttering my home, reducing my belongings by around fifty per cent. I achieved this by selling items, organising council pick-ups, donating to charities and throwing away what was no longer usable. After sprucing up the house, I sold it and relocated to a more desirable suburb closer to my work in Sydney's North Shore.

At this point in my life, early 2021, I started to spend more time out in natural, high-energy and beautiful environments: sitting by the sea, walking in forests or spending time in the mountains. When meditating and reflecting in silence, words of wisdom and guidance began to flow to me. I collected this wisdom in various journals and applied it to my life. This practice transformed my mindset, helping me to move from an uninspired state to an inspired state, and provided the answers I was searching for.

At one pivotal moment on a hill overlooking the ocean, I had a strong sense in my spirit that working solely in the field of administration and customer service was no longer my path and a change was needed. I decided to take a leap of faith and pursue work that aligned more with my strengths. This included teaching tai chi, writing and creating an online course, as well as launching an inspirational merchandise online store. At the same time, I began learning how to become a successful share trader to supplement my income. After two years of living in the North Shore, I decided to move back into my family home to support my elderly mother and focus on my career.

Today, I am in a career I love, waking up each day inspired by my work as a tai chi instructor, writer and share trader. I am also on track to purchasing my dream home in the near future.

Now, it's your turn…

If you are not already living your dream life, this book can help. This book is a collection of wisdom and ideas of success written over many years, all brought together with the aim of assisting you on the journey of successful, inspirational living.

You hold in your hands the action steps and ideas that helped me to move from a life of just getting by to a life I'd only ever dreamed could be realised. It is my hope and wish that by taking in this book's wisdom and applying it to your own life, you too will embark on a journey to seeing your dearest wishes, visions and dreams become a reality. You may have had the thought that your dream is not possible—you're too old or young or there is too much involved in achieving your dream. But the aim of this book is to help transform your thinking so that you can see that the dream is possible.

Each of the chapters in the book is set out in a roadmap to help you on this journey. First, we'll establish or recall what your dream life looks like. Then, we'll clear the obstacles in your way. Next, you will learn how to organise your goals and schedule, so that you can then take action and remain inspired throughout the whole transformative process.

You may also find yourself beginning to enjoy the journey itself, as you become aware of the beauty that is all around and within you. Make sure to appreciate every moment as you take each step closer to living your highest dream and vision for life.

As you read through the book, have a journal on hand to write down the answers and thoughts you have as you work through each chapter's exercises. Participation in the exercises will help you to bring your dream life into existence, one step at a time.

Let's begin!

CHAPTER 1

DREAM ESTABLISHMENT

The acorn begins its life as a small seed,
but, given time and the right conditions,
it can grow into a great tree.
So too can your dream.
Starting out as a vision and sense of knowing,
with nourishment and perseverance, taking an
action step each day in time,
the dream becomes no longer just a
dream—it becomes a reality.

SMALL BEGINNINGS TO A GREAT DREAM

This book is all about the little steps we take each day to keep the commitments and promises we make to ourselves, which lead to gradual improvements that take place over time. The cumulative effect of those little steps is what builds a beautiful life. All of this begins with you recognising that the way you have been living up untill now needs to improve and it may be time to wish for a better way of living.

Give yourself the permission to dream,
the gift of believing this dream is possible
and the gift of persevering until you see your
dream realised.

A dream will sustain you in your everyday life. It can inspire you to learn what you need to learn or do what you need to do to get through the mundane and hard tasks. When times get tough or challenging, it allows you to know that—somehow, someway—you can one day live the life that matches your spirit and vision. If you have a big dream, don't just immediately dismiss it as too far-fetched. Give your dream, and yourself, a chance. Remember this: you are worthy of your dream, and your dream is possible.

It starts as a small wish, just a little hope that things may improve, but if you dig deeper, you may find a dream that has been buried under years of non-acknowledgment, of denial or of just being busy and distracted—buried under seemingly never-ending to-do lists. As you clear away the mental clutter and the clutter in your environment, you'll start to visualise the dream in even greater detail. Ideas may start to flow, and you may find opportunities in your environment that you couldn't see before. Watch as they take on new meaning.

Be true to the calling of your heart. Nourish your greatest dreams into fruition by spending time each day focusing on them.

Great dreams can become true if you take action steps daily and with discipline.
It's important to apply yourself to achieve the highest possible vision for your life.

Dreams don't just take shape by themselves. They require planning, action and review. I went to a seminar over ten years ago where all the participants were asked to write on a card, "I'm on schedule for financial freedom." I strongly believe that one of the most important foundations of a great life begins with the following affirmation: *"I'm on schedule for achieving my dream. I'm on schedule to achieve my highest potential."*

POT OF GOLD

There is a pot of gold, a great treasure, that awaits
every time you remember your dream
and what you are capable of when you reach
your true potential without allowing fear
to hold you back.

What is your dream? Can you see it and feel it? Is it, for example, to love and be loved? To express your gifts in the highest way? To be of service to the world? Or is it to achieve greater abundance in life so that you will have more to give to others?

Later in this book, you will be guided by many exercises that can help you to realise or remember what your dream is. But it all starts with getting quiet and asking yourself questions such as, *"What skills do I have that can help others in some way?"* We all have something unique we can offer the world and something we secretly yearn for if we had nothing stopping or preventing us.

State often when you visualise your dream, *"Thank you. I'm worthy of this dream."* Now, dig deeper. What parts of your heart have you temporarily closed off or tried to close off because you felt you weren't worthy of a dream or that you would make mistakes. Is there a dream you have put on hold for another time and place? What is a small step you can take towards the dream realisation now?

Take the time to listen
and heed the calling of the heart.
Many don't do this, and they wonder
why their lives
lack direction and meaning.

Once you know what your dream is, there's no reason for delay. There's no reason to put your dreams on hold until one magical day when the conditions will be just perfect to act on this plan. Is there anything you can do today to move closer to living the life of your greatest dream?

What makes your heart sing? It may be being out in nature, quietly reflecting. Or maybe you are at your best in a group setting. The answer to this question can be a great clue as to what your dream truly is. I personally love to be out in natural environments—it is where I can reflect and gain clarity about what is important and what isn't and what priorities I need to focus on.

What is important to you? What would life look like if you were living at a higher level, if you were giving your absolute best in all endeavours? Always ask, *"Am I in alignment with my highest vision of myself, my life and with others?"* Don't sell yourself short. Go after the very best and highest dream for your life.

Step up to who you can be
Step up to the one you know you can be.
Step up despite the naysayers.
Step up despite the fear.

Your dream was given to you for a reason.
It can and shall be realised if you give it a chance.
Every day, see your dream, feel your dream
and, with quiet persistence, keep moving
towards it.

Five years ago, I was working full time in customer service and administration in a job that was only utilising a small proportion of my skill set. My dream was to work in a career that would inspire others and make a difference. I started to visualise this dream, what it would look like and entail, such as waking up inspired each day, teaching tai chi to small groups of people, writing a book, putting together an online course and starting to utilise more of my potential. Now, five years later, I am working in my dream career, and I wake up each day with great enthusiasm as I am doing what I love to do. Now, it's your turn.

Exercise

Please take out your journal and write the answers to the following questions.

1. **Mark your starting point.**

   Look at where you are today. What is your starting point? What habits and routines have brought you here? Where would you like to go from here?

2. **Define your dream.**

   Write down your dream with as much description as possible. For example, if it is to live in a beautiful home, what features does the home have? And what would be its location? Another dream could be to have more time and freedom to do what you love to do or to use and develop your unique gifts and talents to a greater extent than you have been. Could you re-work your schedule to make the above possible?

3. Visualise your dream.

Close your eyes for 5–10 minutes to complete the following exercise. It could change your life.

The crowd is clapping and cheering madly. The speaker is about to introduce you to come up on the stage to give a presentation on your skills. How would you like them to introduce you? What would they say to describe the most successful version of yourself? Think about it and, more importantly, feel what this would be like. Take the time to let this feeling soak in. This is the calling that will lead you towards your dream.

Write down in your journal any ideas and wisdom gained from this visualisation.

4. Ask yourself: what can be?

There are no limits to what can be. Give it your best!

As a final step in this exercise, I want you to think even bigger picture. Look beyond your own gifts in the present moment to think with great creativity and potential about the future. I prefer to do this meditation in nature, but you can do it in whatever environment works best for you.

Sit quietly with your eyes closed for 7 minutes or longer, perhaps using the timer on your phone. Simply ask yourself, *"What can be?"* It is important to be patient in this meditation and simply ask yourself that same question over and over. Soon, you may find that wonderful insights, a glimpse of a great dream or idea, or a new way of inspired living may come to mind. After your meditation, write down any new insights in your journal.

CLARITY OF VISION

Only in quietness and stillness
can the heart see its true reflection
on the calm water of peace,
and gain an inspiring vision for the future.

It is important to set aside some time in your schedule for quiet reflection such as being out in nature. In inspiring environments, great ideas and clarity of vision can arrive.

Each Saturday morning, I travel to my favourite beach and watch as the sun rises over the calm ocean. During my meditation, I often receive important insights into life improvement and how to navigate my way through any challenges I am currently facing. I make sure I always have a journal on hand and write down the insights as they arise.

I believe a great vision is a powerful tool for reversing poor habits. Unless you can see what you are wishing and aiming for, you can fall into the trap of lesser aims, mediocrity or worse.

Integrity is the result of having your vision, goals and actions in alignment. So it is always important to ask yourself, *"Is what I'm about to do in alignment with my highest vision and goals?"*

When did life get so busy that we failed to notice the feeling of the grass beneath our feet, the soft breeze on our skin or the warmth of the sun? It's a mistake to be so preoccupied with all that is going on in our lives that we fail to recognise and cultivate a sense of groundedness.

We were not put here on Earth to *do-do-do*, we were put here to *be-be-do*. I feel that a sense of disconnection with the Earth is the start of discontent. Come back to the truth, a feeling of centredness and connection to Earth and all that is and can be. It is here that you can find clarity and the answers to all that is troubling the mind.

A true vision of one's dream can bring tears to the eyes and great hope to the heart.
For a moment, all doubt is extinguished.
You truly believe this vision is possible.
And this is when the magic begins...

A real dream brings excitement and joy whenever you think about it. And the joy does not wane. If you lose interest or forget about the dream easily, it may not be your destiny to achieve it. Unless we know with clarity what we are aiming for, how do we know when we've achieved it?

You should start the process by thinking about your dream. This will help you establish your goals, which will help you set out a plan of action. In that plan, you should work out the dates by which you need to achieve each step.

Think in practical terms about what it would look like to achieve your dream. For example, what would your income be? How many days a week would you want to work? What are financial milestones you could set to achieve this dream in one year? In five years?

As you achieve a clearer vision of how you would like your life to be, you will begin to notice new opportunities as they come your way.

Aim high

The American politician and motivational speaker Les Brown once said, "Shoot for the moon. Even if you miss, you'll land among the stars." It is important to aim beyond what is easy and what you think you deserve. What is your real dream— the dream you would have if there were no limitations of any kind? The dream you have in your heart should be the one you aim for and the barometer of your success.

You can live a life by design or by impulse. Living a life by design, planned to align with your highest vision and dream, is what creates a meaningful and fulfilled life. Consistent and persistent action towards your dream is what helps to bring the dream about.

Exercise

1. Be out in nature.
Set some time in your schedule to be out in nature. For example, being by the sea can be calming for the emotions; hiking

mountains can help build strength, wisdom and reflection; and walking in a forest can cleanse you of negativity and help you to move into a more empowered state.

Once you're there, close your eyes and practise just being in the moment. You may like to place a timer on for 10 minutes. Check at the beginning of the meditation that you have great posture and are practising deep abdominal breathing, not shallow breathing from your upper chest.

Once you've reached a state of inner calm, ponder a challenging situation you are facing and make a wish for clarity. As you reflect upon the challenges, see if any new ideas or vision for your next action come into view. Write down possible solutions.

2. Check for alignment.

Check if your vision, goals and plan of action are all in alignment, and determine if any changes are required. For example, your vision may be to reach a desired fitness level so you can look and feel outstanding. It's important that you know what this would look like; you may like to cut out a picture from a health magazine for inspiration.

A goal along these lines could be a statement that, by the end of the year, you will have reached your ideal body shape by exercising every day and learning about best practices for nutrition.

An action plan may be that every morning for 40 minutes at 6am, you will work out on your bike and do sit-ups and push-ups. On weekends, you will read a health book for half an hour to learn new ideas to implement. This is an action that has worked for me personally. On Saturday afternoons, sitting in my favourite recliner with a warm cup of tea, I have read health books and learned new and wonderful recipes that have improved my diet. Not only has this practice improved my overall wellbeing, but it has drastically reduced my desire to eat out, which has had the further benefit of helping to increase my savings.

3. Highest Life Goals.

Grab a piece of lined paper and write on the top "Highest Life Goals". At the beginning of each line, draw an open box—you'll tick this later, when you've completed the corresponding task. Write down everything you would like to achieve. For example, a goal may be, *"I have now minimised clutter in my home and have only the essential things I really need or that I love. Achieved by* [insert your goal completion date]." or *"I have a budget I will stick to from now until* [date]." Place this in a journal with a tab (so you can find it easily), or you may prefer to type and print it and carry it with you wherever you go. Or you can place it on a wall and look at it every day.

4. Clarity exercise.

If there's an area of your life you would like more clarity in, I recommend the following exercise.

Set your timer for 20 minutes and sit down, with your back upright, straight and supported. With deep and relaxed breathing, meditate on the issue.

For example, the following questions may help you gain clarity about your career. After each question open your eyes to record your answers.

- *What career would I love to be in if there were no obstacles of time or money?*
- *What do I believe is my highest potential in this area of life?*

- *What do I consider to be my purpose?*
- *How can I use my skills and gifts to serve others better?*
- *What would an ideal week in this career look like?*

The next step is to work out a plan of action for how to achieve your vision. Break up your dream into smaller, more manageable tasks. Write down these tasks in your diary. You will find your action steps will naturally be inspired by your new sense of direction.

5. Obtain clarity of purpose.

Without clarity of purpose and meaning, it's easy to be confused about which is the best path to take in life and to be swayed by distractions. For example, if I have nothing planned to action in the day ahead, very little gets accomplished. So, even on my day off, I will purposefully plan my day, which may include reading a book that can assist in my life in some way, or walking out in nature, which will give me time to think and reflect on life.

Here are some questions that can help you to develop clarity of purpose:

- *What is the highest vision I hold for myself and my way of life? Am I in alignment with this?*
- *What exactly am I aiming for in my life?*
- *How can I make something beautiful in my life?*
- *What are three things I would like to achieve this year that are absolute musts for me?*

*When you feel, with every fibre of your being, what
you are truly aiming for, the daily action steps
won't feel so hard to achieve, because you know
where your true destination is.*

6. Imagine your dream.

Imagine your dream, right down to the finest details, as often
as possible. Soon, this dream will become very familiar to you,
and you may gain some insights into how to bring this dream
into reality. For example, to assist with imagining your dream
vacation, you could obtain a brochure from a travel agency for
the place you wish to visit or print out the destination photos
from your research. Each day, visualise being at this destination and enjoying the vacation. Soon ideas may arise as to how
this could become a reality.

You may like to do this as an add-on after your 10-minute
morning meditation. For 5 minutes, imagine or visualise your
dream achieved. I like to visualise the next step in my business
as if it were accomplished. This helps me to develop momentum for working out the next action steps.

7. Set a timeframe for your goal.

Write your goal on a card. Underneath it, write, "*I commit to
achieving this by…*" and write down a date by which the goal
should be achieved. Next, write down the steps you can take
towards it.

For example:

I am so happy that my house is now very organised and clean and that I only have what I

need—items that are useful or hold meaning or that I find beautiful. The rest of the items I have either given away, sold or discarded. I will spend at least 40 minutes twice a week to sort through household items, concentrating on one area of my home until completed. And I will clean the house for 3 hours each weekend. I commit to achieving this by 15 December this year.

TOUCH THE DREAM

Reach out and touch the dream:
visit that property you long to buy, have the
courage to talk to the one you admire,
start that new business.
When you see your dream realised, even if it is
in the imagination, you have a greater chance of
bringing it to life.

You don't have to wait until everything is perfect to reach out to your dream. Can you make room in your schedule to visit a place that makes you feel prosperous or abundant? Spending time in these environments may assist with generating ideas for bringing prosperity closer to real life experience. For example, I like to visit the tea rooms where they have chandeliers, fine china teacups and saucers, little teapots and an assortment of carefully arranged sandwiches, scones and sweets. When in this environment, sipping on the beautiful tea, I ponder, *"How can I improve the abundance of prosperity into my life?"* and ideas often flow.

It is worthwhile to save up so you can visit a place like this, somewhere that feels special and memorable.

Exercise

1. Visit a wonderful, luxurious environment.

When you visit the place, begin to observe the richness of atmosphere, and take notice of the ideas that might flow now that you're in a place of abundance and luxury. Write down some ideas about how it could be possible to live this lifestyle.

Let your ideas flow. For example, if you dream of living by the water, visit a beautiful area by the water, then sit down and feel the energy of the area. Allow nature's inspiration to touch your soul.

2. Place a picture.

Obtain a picture of your dream environment or way of being and place it somewhere in your home that you walk past frequently. Every time you walk past the image, state, *"Thank you for making the way to achieve this clearer to me."* Before long, new and inspired ideas may begin to appear about how to bring your dream to life. Become so familiar in your imagination with your dream fulfilment that the path to get there becomes known.

For example, find a photo of yourself in which you have the physique you desire. Or cut out a picture of the type of body shape you wish for from a fitness magazine and put a photo of your face next to it. Every time you walk past this photo, you will be reminded of and encouraged to reach this state of fitness and wellbeing, and ideas will begin to flow about how you can achieve it.

SUCCESS

Success is to be true to what is in your heart, your highest dream and vision.
Success is taking action steps in alignment and congruence, working on the development of your gifts, to be of service to the world and make a difference.

Always determine if the action you are about to take is in alignment with your overall purpose and highest vision. This will help to protect you from travelling off the path of what you are here in this world to do.

True success in life doesn't happen with one magical event. Life is a bit more complicated and involved than this. Even if you win the lottery, purchase the house of your dreams, marry your soulmate and reach your ideal weight, without core beliefs and wisdom, you won't be able to maintain the dream and you may lose direction. This is why it has been said that wisdom is more valuable than gold—without wisdom, the gold can be lost.

Success is not just the achievement of one life-changing event, but a way of living that aims to progressively realise one's highest potential or purpose for living.

Success means making the most of what you have now, not what you hope to have in the future. Success is an ongoing series of choices and daily disciplines or rituals that all work together to assist in living one's best life. And so, for abundance to continue to flow, it is important to look after and make the best of what you currently have.

> *To not develop or use one's gifts to serve others or the world is to live with an emptiness that no amount of money or distraction can fill.*

It is never easy when you know in your heart and mind that you have so much to offer the world to make a difference, but you are held back by perceived obstacles. So often, people believe that their life needs to be wonderfully perfect, with all their dreams achieved, before they can truly let their light shine.

Don't worry if you don't feel successful yet—if your life is not a ten out of ten in every area, just keep on persevering and keep the vision of what you are aiming for alive.

> *Great dreams can come true if you take action steps daily with discipline, applying yourself to achieve the highest vision for your life.*

Even when I was working full-time in a job I didn't particularly enjoy, I made sure I carved out special time in my schedule where I could write in my journal and consider how I could live truer to my highest vision for my life and what steps I could take towards this. Making a start is what counts.

Exercise

1. Definition of success.
Consider the above definition of success. Write down where you are in your journey towards success. Are you taking daily action steps that are aligned with what you define as your vision and unique gifts? Does your current schedule allow time each day to work on what is truly important to you, and do you consider you are making a difference? Or do you need to make small and big changes in your life?

2. What are the success traits required for your dream?
Next, consider who you need to become and the success traits or qualities you need to realise your dream. Write these down in your journal and review them often to work out how they can be incorporate into your life. Some examples of success traits are:

- focus
- positivity
- discipline
- decisiveness
- clarity of mind
- willingness to learn and to apply the learnings
- self-improvement
- faith that dreams can come true.

3. What do you stand for?

This is an essential guiding question of principle. Just like a lighthouse brings light to help the ships be on the correct course, your values can help guide your way. When the storms of life draw near, what will keep you in alignment with your higher values? If you don't know what you stand for, it may be easy to fall for anything. Write down five values in your journal that you believe in.

Here are some values I believe are very important:

- **Health** – This is of vital importance in becoming the best version of yourself, experiencing the best of life and weathering any storms.

- **Clarity** – To see clearly what the most important action is in each moment of time.

- **Discernmen**t – To see the fine details of the truth; this can protect you from being misled.

- **Inner guidance** – To connect to inner wisdom by spending time in silence. To be aware and in tune with which is the correct path to take in life.

- **Strength** – This can be of great help in challenging times and can be developed in quiet times of reflection, meditation and also through practising martial arts.

Now, write down how these values can be applied to your life. For example:

- *I value wisdom and aim to read something new to develop my skill set for half an hour a day.*

- *I am working in a career in alignment with my highest vision for myself and life.*
- *I'm in the best shape I have ever been in, with excellent energy levels, assisted by disciplined practices of qigong and tai chi and an excellent diet.*

FOUNDATION FOR YOUR DREAM

To build a great structure, you must start with a good base. Something solid but simple. You need a great vision, dream, plan and steps you can action right away—simple, easy steps that can lead you on the road to success.

Take a moment to assess your current skill set and identify areas that may need further development to help you progress towards your dream. The skills you focus on will depend on what you aim to achieve. For example, if your goal is to improve your financial management, are you dedicating time to learning from experts in the field and expanding your knowledge?

I've found that making small, consistent efforts to enhance my skill set each day leads to significant improvements over time. For example, dedicating thirty minutes daily to reading books on business skills has greatly supported me in creating an online course and identifying the best next steps for marketing.

Consider what new skill you can begin that may help you with achieving your vision and dream?

Exercise

Write in your journal how you can allocate time each day to work on the new skill you wish to develop? Then schedule this time in your diary or planner. Even if you can only allocate half an hour a day due to your current commitments, over time, this will add up to some great progress made towards your dream.

CHECK IF YOUR GOALS STRETCH YOU

To state it plainly, goals that are set too low or within a very achievable range, or that are not specific enough, will not have enough motivating power to encourage you through the mundane tasks that you need to complete every day.

It's too vague to simply to have a goal to "do better" in an area of life. I have a friend who, when asked about their goals for the next six months, simply replied, "To improve in business and have a few more clients." They were not specific and did not write their goals down. Although they seem happy, I have noticed they are not making much progress.

As we've seen in previous exercises, it's important to have a vision of what your heart yearns for and to then write it down with some stepping-stone goals that will stretch you and help you to become more than you thought you could become.

To keep you on track, you'll need to review your tasks on a yearly, monthly, weekly and even daily basis and measure your progress. This will help you to determine if the strategy to achieve your goals needs to be adjusted. It's the small adjustments in our daily habits that enable us to stretch in subtle ways, ultimately expanding the horizons of who we can become.

Check if your dreams stretch you and are specific. Make changes if required. For example, if your goal was previously, "*I aim to improve my business income this year*", it can be improved to something like, "*Every evening from 7pm to 8pm, I work out specific ways I can build my marketing and sales skills and improve my yearly income by ten per cent.*"

THE OFFICE WINDOW: CULTIVATING MOTIVATION FOR YOUR DREAM

Have you ever glanced up to look outside your office window, to take one glimpse of the beautiful blue sky, the trees in the distance, and found yourself longing for the big outdoors?

Were we really designed to sit behind a computer all day long and then go home to cook and try to rejuvenate overnight, only to go back and do the eight-hour workday all over again? It may be easy to get caught up in our immediate financial needs, but there is a way out.

It starts with knowing that there must be more to life than this. There is more to life than living like a caged animal, looking out the window for a glimpse of what could be ours if we only had the courage to step out in faith, step up to the person we were created to be and give ourselves a chance to say yes to our own potential and gifts within.

For many years, I endured my mediocre administration job as I could not see any other options at the time. During my lunch break, I would eagerly step out of the office and walk around the building and simply wish for and imagine what my life could be like if I worked for myself instead of on my workplace's goals. I would sometimes sit in a nearby park and visualise this lifestyle.

Eventually, I requested to work four days a week, and, on my free day I would focus on share trading and my writing. Then, one day, I decided to take the leap and give up my four-day role to work full time as a tai chi instructor, share trader, writer and course coach. Each day, I wake up with great enthusiasm as I am now working in a career I love.

Exercise

Take a few minutes to contemplate if there are any areas of life you feel a little stuck in, such as working in a job where you find yourself looking out the window wishing for freedom.

Now, based on some of the exercises we've already completed in this book, review again your dream life and the new skills or actions you could implement to get you there. Now that you've clarified to yourself what your dream is, it's important to start to work out how to bring it into reality.

CHECK IF ASSOCIATIONS ARE SUPPORTIVE

Take a chance on your dream, the glimmer of hope and light that shines through the darkness, making the way clear. You are worthy of your dream. Don't allow others to tell you differently or to somehow steal your confidence. You can make it. You really can.

One of the first key steps to successful living is to assess if the people you spend time with are supportive or non-supportive. They may not share your vision for your dream, but as you make positive changes and they notice you becoming happier and more at peace, they can grow to understand and encourage your journey.

But, if you find you have no one who is supportive of your dream in your immediate environment, consider joining a group of like-minded people, for example, a new exercise group or business group of people who are all motivated to achieve great results in life.

Take a good, honest look at the relationships in your life. Are they supportive in helping you grow into the person you wish to be, or are you just tolerating them? It is a good idea to spend less time with those who you feel are a drain on your energy and start seeking out those who uplift you or who you would love to be more like.

As a single person without a partner to support my goals, I sought inspiration from teachers on YouTube and by attending events like life-improvement courses and networking groups, where I could be surrounded by people striving to better their lives and achieve their goals.

I have reduced time spent with friends who have no drive to improve their lives and am currently developing new friendships with people who have a vision for their lives and are taking steps to realise their vision. As the saying goes, iron sharpens iron. It is always good for us to check our associations.

When it comes to choosing a life partner, I believe a true partner is someone who you can be your authentic self around and someone you don't need to compromise who you truly are for. They are someone who will support you to reach the heights of true potential.

A true partnership happens when two whole people come together—not two people looking to the other to fulfil them somehow. However, partnership is also about each partner helping the other to become the best version of themselves that they can be.

Exercise

Reflect on the above questions and determine if you can make any improvements to your relationships.

Are there any new groups you would like to be a part of that would help develop your skill set in alignment with your dream or new goals? What new action can you take towards achieving your dream?

Even if there is no one you can connect with in your immediate environment, you can start watching inspiring videos on YouTube, listening to podcasts or reading books by those you look up to. This will give you new ways to learn and be inspired.

CHECK YOUR RESOURCES FOR THE JOURNEY

You can't climb Mount Everest if you're wearing only thongs on your feet. And you can't reach your dream without being realistic about the resources and tools that will help get you to your destination.

Assess what resources you have that could be useful for your journey. What physical things might you need to accomplish your dream? Take initiative to account for the physical aspects such as shelter, food, clothing and income that shape the parameters of your life. Only once you do this can you start aiming for your higher accomplishments. Resources like money, books, access to information through internet research or libraries, relationships with successful individuals and time are all valuable assets.

Time is one of our most valuable resources. Do you require more time in your schedule to pursue your dream? Take a look at your current schedule to see if anything can be eliminated or reduced, freeing up precious time to focus on more meaningful pursuits, such as studying strategies for excelling in your career.

I do not own a television for the reason above; I would rather spend time researching topics I am interested in and learning how to improve myself than wastefully watching and listening to news or information that is not in alignment with my aims and dreams.

Exercise

Make a list of possible resources you may need to help you achieve your dream and then ways you can gather them together. For example, to pursue your dream career role in six months' time, what resources will you need? What kind of savings or new skills will be required?

BELIEFS

Great dreams can come true if you truly believe.
Step by step, you can make it.
Believe in yourself and your dream.

Without true belief in what could be possible, we lack the inspiration to take the required actions to bring about the life of our dreams. It all starts with belief. The way to achieve the dream will follow, and then the next step forward will become known.

It is important to be careful about what you hold to be true in your mind—your beliefs about yourself and the world around you. Your beliefs have a huge impact on your actions, and your actions are reflected back in life's circumstances. For this reason, it is wise to always have beliefs grounded in reality.

There are some beliefs that can hold you back. Some people believe that they are better than others, have some great spiritual power or are entitled to success without effort. These beliefs can hinder genuine connection and personal development.

The truth is that we have all been given a unique and wonderful gift. The key is to work on your unique gift, or set of gifts, and seek to improve upon them every day. If you are not experiencing the level of success that you desire in a certain area, question the beliefs you are currently holding in that area, whether it's finances, business, relationships or your emotional state.

You are beautiful and talented and have a great gift to bring to the world. Don't think for one moment you are not good enough or not equipped to bring your great dream into reality. You have what you need already—take that first step and take it now.

Every day, do something that uplifts the spirit,
makes the soul sing and for one moment in time,
helps you to believe that anything is possible.
Visit this enchanted place often, especially if expe-
riencing any of life's challenges, a place where you
believe there are no limitations, and where you can
be and have whatever you wish for.

A great technique I use to improve my beliefs is to affirm the way I wish them to be. For example, whenever I feel a sense of lack creeping into my consciousness, I affirm, "*I am wealthy beyond measure. I have what it takes to achieve my dreams in all areas of my life.*"

Exercise

1. Write down your beliefs.

Write down the beliefs you currently hold to be true in relation to your health, career, finances, relationships, spirituality and emotions, and then assess if they are supportive of your greatest dreams. If you discover that you are holding any unsupportive beliefs—for example, "*It's too hard to get into good physical shape,*"—why not challenge those beliefs by stating the opposite: "*In time, if I stick to my new workout schedule of 30 minutes of exercise a day, I can be well on the way to reaching my fitness goal.*"

2. Imagine that you've achieved your dream.

Write in your journal the heading "I've made it!!!" Imagining that you've achieved your dream, complete the following sentences:

- I'm a successful…
- I've reached my…
- I've purchased…

For example:

- I'm a successful business owner and I can now set my own schedule.
- I've reached my ideal body shape: trim and toned.
- I've purchased my new home.

Write a date for each by which you need to achieve the goal. Review this daily or at least once a week.

DREAM FULFILMENT

Believe you are enough and that you have what you need to fulfil your destiny.

I used to think that, at a special time and place, my greatest dreams would come true. For a very long time, I believed that I had to secure financial independence (where assets bring in more income than is required for expenses) before I could share my true gifts with the world. But one day, in quiet meditation, I realised there was another way. I started to generate a new belief. I said to myself, *"My gifts will make a way for me. Sharing them is the key to living a successful life. There is nothing honourable about holding back your gifts from the world."*

Living with true purpose, joy and fulfilment is all about working on what you are called to do in this world. Don't just be a dreamer, wishing and hoping your dreams will come true. Work on the development and refinement of your skill set to align with your true gifts and talents. Working on and refining your skills can set you on the pathway to achieving your dream.

Never forget this important truth: achieving one dream can help create momentum for more dreams to be achieved. Taking stock of the dreams that have already come true in your life will help you to generate an understanding of what it takes for even more dreams to come true.

When I reflect on my life, I'm able to see that I've achieved some great dreams. As mentioned earlier, at twenty-one, after practising karate for many years, I became a world champion and performed a second dan kata. Another dream was buying a home. After careful budgeting and saving for over seven years, I was able to buy a home in 2011. A third dream that has come true is that I have raised, as a single parent, a beautiful girl who is generous and kind and who is achieving outstanding things with her life.

Exercise

Reflect on the dreams you've already achieved in your life. Can some of the skills obtained from these achievements be of assistance with your current dreams and goals?

CHAPTER 2

CLEARING THE WAY

A calm lake can show clear reflections. So too can a calm state of mind produce a clear vision of what is important.

By freeing the heart, mind and environment of all unnecessary clutter, one begins to see the true reality of what is, what can be, and what one is truly capable of.

Freedom occurs when we unburden ourselves from all that is unnecessary and work towards that which is necessary.

NEW DAY

Each new day is a gift.
How often do we stop and appreciate all we have
and the beauty of each moment?

E ach morning is a new day, a new start. Release the baggage of all the unfulfilled dreams, past mistakes and failures. Say to yourself, *"I'm going to give my dreams a chance to see the light of day. I'm worthy of success. I'm going to take some action today. No matter how small, I'm going to make progress."*

It's important to believe that you have what it takes to be successful. Without the belief, you may unintentionally fill up your life with just survival mentality and clutter, or, worse, you may substitute your dream with what was not meant to be. When you have true belief in yourself and your dream, you can start taking inspired action towards achieving it. It all begins by starting the day with true appreciation of this very moment and treating each day as a new beginning and opportunity to start again.

SPACE CLEARING—MAKING WAY FOR THE NEW.

At one stage, I was living in a house cluttered with unused furniture and belongings; I was working full time in a job that was unfulfilling, to put it mildly; and I was residing in a sub-urb that failed to inspire me.

Gradually, I began to remove all that was not necessary or essential, and I kept only things that brought me peace or happiness. I believe that the more clutter you clear away the more you can see clearly what is important.

After three council pickups of old furniture, selling items online and donating many bags of clothing to charity, my home began to feel much more spacious, and I began to experience greater clarity in my mind and about the new direction I wanted to take.

After having the walls repainted, installing new blinds and completing the landscaping, I put the house on the market. It sold within a month, allowing me to start a new chapter of my life in a more minimalistic home located in an inspiring area.

Environment does affect us, either positively or negatively.

You don't reach the top of a mountain in a single step. Gradual progress is what gets you there. Keep your eye on the summit and eliminate distractions. The same principle applies to clearing clutter.

Aim to focus on at least one area of your home every week. For example, the pantry. In a well-organised pantry, just one glance can reveal what you have. This is very useful for menu planning.

Many believe that acquiring new things will make them happier, but it's only when you let go of all that is superficial and no longer serving the person you aspire to be that happiness and abundance can begin to emerge. Notice the beauty in nature, and see if you can make your home also a place of beauty and peace—a haven for the body, mind and soul.

Exercise

Work out a plan of action for decluttering your home. Divide the space into distinct areas. For example, declutter the clothes in the closet and then the clothes in the drawers rather than trying to tackle everything at one time. This can help prevent overwhelm.

Start by decluttering for only 40 minutes a week, but, once you see progress, you may want to increase this duration. You can enlist the help of others to assist in determining what is truly needed and useful.

Keep a list of all the areas you have decluttered. Over time, you will feel a great sense of accomplishment as you reflect on how far you have come.

TAKE STOCK OF WHAT YOU HAVE

Make sure you have a good look at what you already have that can be utilised for the realisation of your dreams. Clear anything that isn't meaningful to you. With the vacuum created, you then allow good things to come into your life. Create the space to attract what you wish for.

I love reading and enjoy buying new books, but, before purchasing a new one, I take a moment to reflect on the ones I already own. I ask myself, *"Have I read all the books I currently have, and have I truly understood and applied their wisdom to my life?"* This helps me reassess and appreciate my collection, often leading me to revisit important books that can make a difference in my life. When re-reading, I take notes along the way and complete any recommended exercises, instead of skimming through. This way, my understanding grows, and I can more effectively apply the book's insights to improve my life.

However, if I come across a book that I believe will offer new wisdom or valuable insights beyond what I currently possess, I make the decision to purchase it, knowing it will contribute to my growth and learning.

Exercise

Look around your home and assess what you have already. Look in kitchen cupboards, in the fridge and around your office. Determine if any of these areas need to be refined, organised or utilised better.

PLUG THE LEAKS IN THE BOAT

Just like a boat can sink if there is a large leak, you can find yourself underwater if you have financial leaks caused by unnecessary spending habits. There are many valuable resources to help you save money, such as books on budgeting and living frugally, but a simple thing you can do is evaluate if there are any financial leaks in your spending and calculate how much they are costing. For example, some people like to buy new things to lift their mood when they're feeling down; however, these purchases are often not necessary. Before buying something, it can be helpful to ask yourself, *"Do I really need this?"* and, *"Does this align with my higher values and goals?"*

By plugging these leaks, you can accelerate the timeline for realising your dreams. My biggest tip for living frugally and economically is to cook for yourself at home instead of eating out. Can you grow your own vegetables or learn cooking skills? It's easy to find recipes online or in books— try second-hand shops or borrow them from the library.

My mum said once, "If you know how to read, you can cook." Just like learning anything new, teaching yourself to cook may stretch you beyond your comfort zone at the start. But, if you keep persisting, you will eventually become proficient. My nephew, who always relied on his mother for meals growing up, turned to YouTube for cooking lessons when he moved out. Now, he cooks quite well. Start by trying out one new recipe each week. See which ones you enjoy and consider adding them to your regular meal rotation.

How far are you prepared to go to make room for your dreams? How much could you save if you cut out all unnecessary spending and splashed out only on special occasions? Have you considered the impact this could have? I have discovered that I would much rather save up for a beautiful fine-dining experience that I enjoy and savour as a rare treat than buy takeaway on a regular basis. I am often amazed how much can be saved just by taking the time to be more organised and to prepare food at home instead of eating out often.

REST AND REPRIEVE

Rest can rejuvenate and re-energise you at different stages in your journey towards achieving your dreams. When is the last time you rested on soft grass next to a beautiful stream of water? Sometimes, the best ideas arrive when we are the most relaxed. Rest gives you the energy and rejuvenation to keep striving for your dream achievement.

I personally use Saturdays as my day of rest. Rather than using this day for extensive planning or activities, I leave it as a blank canvas—as a day to dream, learn and meditate. As I meditate, whether out in nature or at home, I often receive insights about parts of my life that need to change for me to move closer to my highest vision. I also use my day of rest to learn new practices for enhancing health and wellbeing by reading excellent health-related books. Practising tai chi and qigong further helps to revitalise and refresh my body, mind and spirit.

Many traditions and cultures advocate for a weekly day of rest, often on a Saturday or Sunday. Allow time in your schedule for rest and rejuvenation. If a full day of rest isn't feasible, could you at least set aside half a day? On your day (or half a day) of rest, remember to carry a notebook with you so that you can record new insights and ideas for life improvement.

Exercise

Take a look at your calendar. Once all your work and other important activities have been scheduled, can you find a 4-hour window available to use as your time of rest? Block out this time for rest, rejuvenation and life reflection.

CULTIVATING DISCIPLINE

Excellence with discipline and habits helps to bring about excellence in life.

Cultivating discipline in life begins with being the gatekeeper of your thoughts, as what we dwell on can open the gate to what we experience. Discipline can also be developed through firm self-questioning. Consider asking yourself some of the following questions:

- *How long can I live in denial of my greatest gifts to the world?*
- *I long for a great abundance and richness of being and doing, but how can this be achieved if I'm settling for mediocrity and laziness?*
- *I say I want to be wealthier, but am I saving and investing all I can?*
- *I say I want to be healthier, but am I exercising regularly and doing all I can to have an excellent diet?*
- *I say I would like to experience love, but am I taking chances to meet people or stepping out of my comfort zone?*

There is a time and place for rest and feeling peace and joy, but too much will get in the way of your quest for your dream achievement. Your schedule should have pockets of time for rejuvenation and rest but mostly cater for study, work, development and refinement of gifts, house cleaning and maintenance, and exercise. This balance will work wonders to help you achieve your greatest dreams. A schedule that is heavily focused on easy activities like relaxation, watching TV, excessive takeaway and going out can do more harm than good in the pursuit of realising one's potential and purpose.

Ask, *"How can I obtain the fuel to propel my dreams into reality?"* Examples of good fuel include regular exercise, an excellent diet and education in your field of interest. All these elements can work together wonderfully to give you the necessary energy to bring your dreams into reality.

Imagine that you're ninety and are having the following realisation: *"I am not living the life I dreamed about, when I was young, because I was too lazy. I indulged in all that was superficial and meaningless and wasted precious time when I should have been disciplined and developed my gifts so that I could bring something of value to the world."*

You want to be able to look in the mirror and say, *"Yes, I am really doing and being all I can to realise my highest potential and dream. I am not here just to have a good time but to make something wonderful, beautiful and useful of my life, gifts and time."*

An effective tool for cultivating discipline is a *Time Tracker*. It's essentially a piece of paper with the date at the top and a vertical line down the centre. The left-hand column is Time; the right-hand column is Scheduled Activities. Each night, in the Scheduled Activities column, I list my goals for the next day, and, beside them on the left, I write specific times, typically in forty-minute intervals (with twenty-minute breaks to exercise or rest). As I complete each task, I mark it with a tick. For example, from 5am to 5.40am, I might schedule time for studying new marketing techniques for my business. After finishing, I would tick it off as done. This brings a sense of accomplishment at the conclusion of each day, as I can look at the time tracker and see that I have completed all of my planned activities.

TIME TRACKER 15 April	
Time	**Scheduled Activities**
5am–5.40am	Study new marketing techniques
5.40am–6am	Light exercise and stretching
6am–6.40am	Review goals and meditate

Exercise

Take a look at your schedule of activities from the last week and consider how much time was spent in activities that are in alignment with what is truly important and that required discipline. Consider if you are content with your current schedule or if you need to make improvements.

A useful tool to keep you on track (along with a Time Tracker) is a *Habit Tracker*. This is a piece of paper that lists 3 to 4 habits you'd like to cultivate down the left side and the days of the week across the top, with a tick box for each habit, each day. Tick the box if you've completed the habit each day. At the end of each week, you can assess if any improvements are required. You may also like to research what is available online to help you keep track of habits, such as an app on your phone.

LEARN TO SAY NO

It is important to learn to say no to anything that is not in alignment with your highest goals. This includes resisting the temptation to do what's easy in the moment if it takes you off the path you're meant to follow.

Learn to say no.
No to bad habits.
No to clutter.
No to being inauthentic.
If you give in all the time, how can you create the
space for anything good in your life?
Learn to say no to what does not hold real meaning.
Give your life the chance to be outstanding.

It is sad to give up or let go of things or relationships you once held dear. It can be difficult, but, when they no longer align with your higher values, it's sometimes necessary to let go of the good to make way for the great.

You cannot settle in the valley if it is the mountain-
top you aspire to reach.

There was a stage in my life where I felt in my spirit that "average" or "good enough" was no longer okay. I couldn't allow the next ten years of my life to be like the previous ten years. I decided to hold myself to a higher standard and vision.

Reviewing my goals on a daily basis helped me to say no to other demands on my time that were not in alignment. If I hadn't done this and worked on things that were of low importance or not in alignment, I would not be where I am today.

Exercise

At the conclusion of each week, evaluate if there is any excess that needs to be reduced or eliminated to allow more space for your goals.

At the conclusion of each year, create a list of all the habits you would like to leave behind before you step into the new year. You can call the list "What I am leaving behind in the current year". For example, it may be procrastination on starting your new business or laziness in not sticking to your exercise plan. You can then tear apart the list and throw it in the bin, releasing attachments to any negativity.

SELF-WORTH

Be true
to your greatest dream
in thoughts,
in words,
in actions.
Congruence in all things
helps with the momentum, strength and
nourishment required
for the realisation of your dream.

So many people in today's world suffer from low self-esteem and low self-worth. If someone views themselves as not worthy of great love and abundance, how can they achieve it?

A great minister once said, "He or she who feels most forgiven feels the most blessed." We must forgive ourselves for all our past mistakes, so they don't rob us of our future. Each person lives according to what they believe is possible for them. Let go of low self-worth; you are worthy of great things. You're a valuable person.

Be on guard for negative thoughts or emotions. At all times, you have the power to gently change your mental focus to more empowering thoughts. Even the music we listen to can affect our mental state. This is perhaps why I like listening to classical and meditation music so much. As there are no lyrics, I can concentrate much better on asking empowering questions and focusing on what is important. I was surprised to learn that the words that you listen to are like affirmations. Is what the artist is singing about something you would like to affirm in your life?

Exercise

In your weekly review time, such as on a Sunday evening, determine if there are any areas of your life requiring forgiveness for yourself or others. You can write this down in your journal. What could be possible for you?

Assess what voices and music you are currently allowing to speak into your life and if any changes are needed.

LETTING GO OF REGRET

*It's only a mistake if you haven't learned
the lesson.*

In 2017, I wrote a phrase in my journal that summed up the concept of letting go of regret, inspired by a motivational talk I had listened to online: *"It is not how many years lost or wasted but how many years you have left to make a difference that is important now."*

Reflecting on the many years I spent in a career that was not aligned with my true skills and gifts, and how long it took me to finally have to the courage to pursue what I truly love, it would be easy to fall into the trap of feeling negativity or regret. But I have learned that we only have what is in our lives in the present moment. Dwelling on what we should have achieved already or on past inaction or unfairness only generates sadness and regret.

It may be tempting to get caught up in thinking, *"If only I could have met my dream soulmate, I could have avoided starting wrong relationships,"* or, *"If only I had worked out a plan and taken action on my dream life sooner, I would have avoided years of unfulfilling work and sadness."* But this foundation doesn't support a fulfilling future. There comes a time when you must release the sadness and regret and have the courage to let go of the old feelings to make room for a new way of living and being.

Here are some ways to let go of regret and nourish your dream life:

- Move into a high-energy state. This is a state in which you feel wonderful and positive about your life and possibilities for the future, just like you would feel after a great workout at the gym. An effective way to achieve this is by focusing on good posture and excellent breathing habits to let out all the negative feelings and allow in the good feelings.

- Clear clutter that may be related to unsupportive memories.

- Visit high-energy, beautiful areas that will encourage higher levels of thinking, feeling and generating vision.

- Review your goals, plans and dreams for the future often.

- Maintain a clean home: freshly vacuumed and dusted and with all the washing done. The home can foster renewal and act as a springboard to goal achievement.

It is important to reach a place that allows you to see yourself as truly valuable and truly forgiven for past mistakes and to recognise the gifts you have to help make the world a better place. *Could've, should've, would've*—these are the words of regret. Let the past rest in peace, because we only have what is here and now.

Exercise

1. Regret balloon.

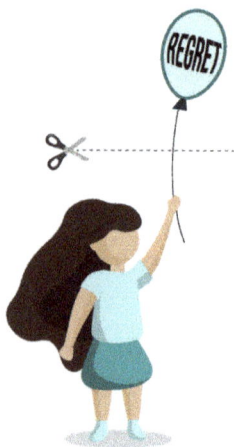

Close your eyes and imagine you are holding a balloon. Blow into the balloon any regret you have been holding on to and then tie up the balloon. Now, imagine a pair of scissors cutting the string that holds it to you.

Release the balloon and state, *"I now release any regret I have been holding on to, in love and light."* Now, breathe in the qualities you would like more of, such as courage, strength and abundance.

2. Letting go of excess baggage.

For many years, I carried excess baggage. I had too many things that didn't add value to my life. This clutter left me feeling stuck. However, once I started clearing and eliminating it, I felt lighter and more equipped to make some major improvements in my life.

Make a list of what is currently weighing you down. This could be physical clutter, emotional burdens or habits that hinder your progress towards achieving your goals. Examples might be an unhealthy diet, lack of regular exercise, spending beyond your budget or struggling with procrastination and lack of motivation.

Now, beside each, write what this baggage is costing you. For example, feeling insecure can cost you the confidence that you need to pursue your dream.

Write down possible strategies on how you can release this baggage and create something new in its place. For example, if you're feeling insecure about a particular skill set, what can you study for half an hour a day that can help improve your skills?

TRANSFORMING DOUBT

Stretch
Don't doubt your dream or water it down
with something you think is more achievable.
Stretch yourself.
Strive forward.
We don't make progress by having weak goals.

Move back into alignment with your inner truth and joy. Let joy—not doubt—be your compass guiding you towards your path. When others challenge you about your decisions, speak your truth quietly and clearly from the heart. Be assertive in standing up for your values, remembering that no-one knows you better than you know yourself.

It is also important not to allow other people's words of doubt about your abilities affect you. Let me share a personal example. A few months before my dad passed away, my sister filmed a video of him sharing messages for each of his daughters. He had encouraging words for my sisters, but, when it came to me, he said, "Catherine has all these dreams, but I don't think she'll bring them about in life." Initially, this was disappointing, but it led me to a realisation: it's my job to believe in myself, no one else's. This inspired me to create a quote for my Redbubble store, *GlimmeringDream*: "It is my job to believe in me, no one else's!" and another one, "Know your value and the value you bring to the world."

Yes, life may present obstacles and sway you temporarily, but think of yourself like a palm tree: flexible in the wind yet always returning to your centre. If you remain steadfast in your dream, the wind will pass and you can gather your resources to nurture and bring your dream into realisation.

Trying to please everyone is not possible. The secret to success is to know your true heart's song and live out this song by the way you live your life. There is a part of you that says yes to life, yes to abundance, yes to being the best you can be. So surround yourself with people who will do the same and support your dreams. When others see how happy you are for taking a chance on your dream, they may also find the courage to take a chance on their dream. Be around people who uplift your spirit and encourage you to rise to your full potential.

Exercise

Evaluate if those in your company are an inspiration to you. Do they encourage you to be your best? Or do they do the opposite? Being able to discern the truth in this matter is a valuable gift.

CREATING ABUNDANCE

Abundance is all around.
You just need to notice it.
There is not just one blade of grass,
not just one flower.
Welcome abundance in your life;
you are worthy of it.

Once you feel you have cleared your inner and outer environment, allow yourself to dream. Listen to words of inspiration and encouragement, such as from inspirational speakers on YouTube. Start to feel deserving of your dream and abundance in life.

Abundance is the opposite of scarcity. While scarcity is rooted in the belief that there is never enough—whether that be money, time, love or opportunities—abundance embraces the mindset that there is more than enough to go around. It is also the state of recognising the wealth of resources, connections and possibilities already present in your life.

Along with listening to inspiring words on abundant living from great speakers, start to listen to the words you say to yourself. Pay close attention and challenge them when you notice they stem from a mindset of scarcity, such as thoughts of lack, fear or self-doubt. Shift your focus to gratitude and potential, affirming that your dreams are possible and within reach.

Let go of scarcity from your system and create a life of abundance.

Keep track of what is important to you to prevent unnecessary loss and to help you generate abundance in your life. For example, creating a budget and tracking your expenses can help you take control of your finances and allocate money towards what truly matters, rather than wondering where it went. However, it's important not to dwell on past financial mistakes or lost funds. Instead, focus on using awareness of where your money is going as a tool to make more intentional choices moving forward, reinforcing a mindset of growth and abundance.

Drawing greater abundance to your life starts with noticing the abundance already present. What we focus on expands. Be in the driver's seat of your life. Are you allowing circumstances to dictate how you feel, or are you deciding how to feel and what to experience? You should decide first how you wish to feel and then adjust your actions accordingly to generate more of this feeling. If you wish to feel more abundance instead of what you are lacking, consider what you are already grateful for and notice abundance all around in nature; then, you may draw more abundance towards you.

While wishing for greater abundance in life is wonderful, take this precautionary note. While it is great to strive for accomplishments and want to be better, continuously wanting more and more can only make one feel empty.

Are you truly appreciative of all you have now? Be happy now. Be peaceful now. Happily and peacefully work towards achieving your dreams.

Make a difference

Abundance in feeling comes not from what we get or take from the world, but from what we can give to the world that truly makes a difference. You don't have to wait until everything in your life is perfect before you make a difference. What can you do today to make someone's day shine brighter? I like to bring a gift when I visit someone, and, if I don't have a gift, I prepare a compliment. I have found this brightens my day just as much as it brightens the day of the person receiving it.

Exercise

Start by noticing where you already have abundance in your life. For example, having excellent health and great relationships is a form of abundance. Each day, say a prayer of gratitude for the abundance you are becoming more aware of, especially at times you start to notice any feelings of lack.

Also, if your schedule allows, spend some time in nature, such as in a botanical garden. Look around and notice the great abundance present. Notice all the beautiful flowers in the rose garden.

REMEMBER THE DREAM

It is of great importance to remember the dream. The dream is what can keep you going and continuing to take action when times get tough. Remembering your true dream will help you take only those actions that are in alignment with your highest values and intentions.

If you don't know the dream, it can be easy to get distracted or fill your life with lesser concerns and unsupportive people. This is how excess and clutter can arise. We think we want one thing but will settle for something else if the dream is not strong enough.

How will your dream come to pass if something else is in its way? Make space for what is most important to you. You are good enough for your greatest dream to be realised. You are valuable. You have something great to contribute to the world. Never again think you're not good enough to be someone who is wonderful and inspiring.

Sometimes, we can believe the discouragement of others. We can be caught in a survival mentality or become too busy and lose sight of the dream and the life we wish to lead. But, to maintain hope in our hearts, it is important to have an inner knowing and a great belief that the dream can be achieved.

Today is a new day to get it right—to start the best actions that will help you nourish your great dream into reality.

CHAPTER 3

ORGANISED POWER

*Just as a sunrise or sunset appears at a specific time,
opportunity may not always be present,
but you can be observant and prepared
for when opportunity does appear.*

*If the dream is strong enough, a way will be found.
We schedule in what is most important to us.*

PREPARE FOR SUCCESS

Preparation is essential for success. A great example is a picnic. I enjoy a carefully prepared picnic so much more than simply eating out. Imagine this: you're sitting on a picnic rug, a delicious and healthy meal rests atop a small picnic table in front of you, and your eyes rest on a calm lake. You see ducks swim by and feel the warmth of the sun and a gentle breeze through the palm trees. In order to have the full experience of the above, and for success in general, good preparation is required.

Another example is planning for the day ahead the night before. This not only prevents wasting time in the morning but also helps immensely with building momentum. Organised plans, put into action, can accomplish so much more than just drifting along.

Don't just skim the surface of
what you're truly capable of.
Start drawing on and developing your
greatest gifts.

If your dream is clear and strong enough, you will find a way to make time for it, no matter how busy your schedule is. Prepare for opportunity, so that, when it comes along, you can reach out with both hands and grab hold of it. It's yours because you are ready for it.

For too long, I hid my talents and gifts from the world. I was waiting for the perfect time when my great dreams of income replacement, an ideal home near the beach and reaching my ideal body shape would all come true. I heard how important it was to live by example. Or, as the motto at my daughter's school put it, "In deed, not word." This reminded me that taking action, even in imperfect circumstances, is far more powerful than waiting for the "right time". I was holding back, thinking I needed to wait until everything fell into place to share my experiences and gifts with others. This mindset only delayed my progress and prevented me from making an impact.

Still, I continued writing and working in the background, trusting that the right opportunities would soon arise. When my dream started to take shape, I realised I didn't need to start from scratch—those small, consistent efforts had already set the stage for success.

You don't need to wait until life is absolutely perfect to start taking action on your dream. I cultivated a new belief, one that has continued to sustain me: *"Developing my gifts and skill set will pave the way to achieving my dream and making a difference in the world."* Your gifts could be the golden ticket you are searching for—a way to make your dreams come true.

There are no excuses for those who are serious about their dream.

Following a dream requires a plan and effort, but it may also require some fine-tuning if your current approach isn't yielding the results you desire. For example, exercising for twenty minutes a day is a great start, but it may not be enough to achieve your desired body shape. You might need to adjust to forty minutes of exercise a day, paired with a healthy and well-balanced diet.

Aim for a little, plan for a little, achieve little. Aim for your highest and biggest dream possible, plan for great things, and what you achieve may be better than your wildest dreams and expectations.

Exercise

1. Journalling prompts.

Take out your journal and write answers to the following questions:

- *How much do you really want your dream?*
- *Are you prepared to put in the effort required?*
- *If you are on the right track for dream achievement, do you just need to ramp up your efforts?*
- *Is a timeframe adjustment needed for some of your goals and dreams?*

2. Binder of vital documents.

Now, it's time to create some order with your dreams, goals and finances. Obtain a binder and place the following inside:

- **Yearly goals** with categories such as health, career, finances, spiritual life, home and relationships. You can add in some pictures you have found online or in magazines that can act as a visual reminder of what you are aiming for.

- **Budget:** income, expenses and savings.
- **Savings calculator** based on estimated savings for years ahead. Also to determine how much you would need to save or generate per month to accomplish your dreams and goals.
- **Costs** associated with following your dream.

* Note: if you are unsure how to create the finances categories, please consult with your accountant or financial planner. Also, there are many valuable resources online and in books.

CHOOSING YOUR SCHEDULE

Structuring your day is the key to bringing a great dream into reality.

When creating your schedule, it is important to prioritise your most important task. Although there are many books and resources on time management, I believe excellent time management begins with deciding what holds the most importance to you and making sure you are allocating time for it accordingly.

In my morning meditation, I ask the question, *"What is important for me to do today?"* If it is not already on my list of goals for the day, I make sure I add it in.

It starts with a dream, followed by a belief that
you can achieve that dream. The next step is to
learn about the best path forward and then to take
action, refine your skills and apply your wisdom.

Choose your schedule with the belief, "*I have what it takes to succeed in all areas of my life.*" Never take for granted the opportunity and possibilities of the present moment. While it is nice to dream of a wonderful future or reminisce about the past, it is important to bring your attention to the now as much as possible. It is in the present moment that you lay the building blocks for this wonderful future.

Step by step, focus on one important task at a time and prioritise excellent scheduling. With excellent preparation and organised power in the area of life aligned to your true calling and gift, you will start to feel an inner knowing that your life's dream is possible. You will feel a great release of energy, peace and joy knowing your gift can truly make a difference in another's life.

Focus, focus, focus. Use time well, for it is a limited resource. A schedule helps to nurture a great dream into reality.

Exercise

Set a timer for 10 minutes with the intention of gaining a clear idea of what your next step needs to be and how you can prepare for it.

Ask, "*What is the best step I can make next for my career?*" (Or you may ask the question for any other area of life you are seeking clarity in.) Open your eyes and write down your answer. Consult your schedule and block in the time required for this next step.

GENERATING THE RESOURCES FOR YOUR DREAM

In what ways can you generate income that are in alignment with your skills, talents and dreams? Together with saving, making the most of what you already have and eliminating unnecessary expenditure, generating another source of income may be very beneficial in giving your dream a big boost.

Ideas include:

- coaching others in the field of your passion
- selling unwanted items around the house
- working part time on your hobby until the hobby generates more income than your job and you can start reducing your work hours.

Decide what you would like to excel in and schedule forty to sixty minutes per day for study in this area.

40 minutes x 365 days per year

= 14,600 minutes/year

= 243.33 hours/year

= 6 weeks of full-time work (40 hours/week) towards your dream

Learning is important, so as not to re-invent the wheel.
Never underestimate the power of learning.
If you're learning, you're growing.

To achieve financial stability and independence, it's essential to commit to daily learning. A wealth of valuable information is readily available through platforms like YouTube, as well as in books and courses, offering endless opportunities to grow your knowledge and skills.

Reading fiction and watching TV can be enjoyable and entertaining, but if you're working towards achieving your dream, it's wise to limit the time you spend on these activities. Instead, prioritise dedicating more of your time to non-fiction and educational resources that can support your growth and help you move closer to your goals—books that will inspire and teach; books from others who have achieved what you want to achieve and who you can learn from.

A guide can only be a guide if they have first walked the trail with success. Seek a mentor who has already achieved what you wish to achieve. Read, listen to and study their works and attend and participate in their conferences and workshops. Along with being organised at home, it is beneficial to be organised with your dreams and finances.

Exercise

Review your schedule and determine what would be the best time to commence your day and the best time for your financial freedom study time. Schedule these times in and commit to actioning them.

MORNING ROUTINE

At the start of the day, I like to do a simple exercise that can be done anywhere—even while driving. I have found it not only generates positive feelings and motivation but also sets an excellent foundation for the day. It's practical too, helping to turn lofty dreams into concrete, actionable steps.

Here it is:

3 x 3 x 3

Think about:

- three things you are **grateful for**,
- three **great wishes** for the future, and
- three **goals** for the day.

This will help bring your big picture wishes into the reality of the present moment.

At the start of the day, instead of focusing on all the things you must do, why not consider what can be? What would you like to create or experience?

For example:

- rejuvenation in nature
- a clean house
- being in excellent physical shape
- increased learning and wisdom through reading.

If you can visualise your goals, the tasks themselves won't feel as daunting.

Wake up early

When I sleep in, I feel sluggish. Getting up early not only gives you time to learn new things, but the early morning is also the most magical time of the day. It is the best time for walking and experiencing nature and the best time to study, because you're at your most mentally alert and focused.

It is always best to do what is hard early in the day, such as exercise and study. My highest energy levels are in the morning, so I make sure to capitalise on this by starting my skill-building exercises or most important tasks between 5am and 6am.

Later in the day, I transition to more enjoyable activities like meditating, reviewing my dreams and goals, and going on a walk. Evaluate where in the day you have the most energy and aim to complete your most challenging tasks at this time.

EVENING ROUTINE

At the conclusion of the day:

- Assess how you went with achieving your daily goals and if any improvements can be made. Give yourself a rating out of ten for how much of your potential you utilised during the day. (A rating of "0" means no potential was utilised, and a "10" means you are happy you did your absolute best in utilising your potential. You may like to further extend this exercise and evaluate your potential utilised in your personal life and then in your business life.)

- Review your calendar and write your main goals for the next day. This way, when you wake up, you can get started right away taking action on your most important and highly valued tasks.

- Remember also to do some stretches for about 10-15 minutes to maintain your flexibility and prevent unnecessary muscular aches or pains.

Before going to sleep:

- Say a **prayer of gratitude**, starting with, *"Thank you for the blessings of today…"*
- Consider the **three best things** that stood out to you today. It could be that first sip of coffee, seeing the sunrise or being around inspiring people.
- Ask yourself, *"What is **one excellent thing** I have learned today?"* We learn something new every day, and it is important to capture and understand these lessons to continue growing and improving.

BUILDING YOUR SKILL SET

Don't just be a dreamer, wishing and hoping your dream will come true.
Develop and refine your skill set in alignment with your true gifts and talents.
When you become outstanding at what you do, dream achievement is not too far away.

Anyone can be successful for one day, but for sustained and increasing success, you need an excellent routine of daily practices that can help you improve in your area of expertise and in becoming better in all other areas of life as well.

Practices, as referred to in this book, are activities you can do that bring about a positive change of state, build inner strength or develop greater resilience, clarity and improved wellbeing. Practices may include expressing gratitude, morning exercise, listening to inspiring teachings while getting ready, reading self-improvement books and tuning in to your inner wisdom during moments of silence and solitude. They can serve as a safety net to provide uplifting support in times of need. So schedule these practices into your daily routine to uplift your spirit and help you with whatever challenges may arise during the day.

When considering what practices to include in your daily routine, consider what area you want to improve in the most. Gaining new skills in an area you find challenging can help you gain confidence. For example, if you find you need to develop your skills in public speaking to assist you in your career growth, there are local organisations and groups, such as Toastmasters, that can assist. There are also great books on this topic you could read to learn more.

Seeking to become excellent at what you do brings about success in your field of endeavours. We are never truly the very best we can be—there is always room for growth. If you believe you are the best you can be at something, there is no growth, only arrogance. A humble attitude brings out the best results because it shows you that there is always room for learning and improvement.

Answer the following:

- *In which areas of my life would building a new set of skills be most beneficial?*
- *How would this contribute to my career growth?*
- *What time can I allocate on my calendar for building this skill set?*

VISION STATEMENT

When you are in an awesome, high-energy state, write a letter to yourself that you can read and refer to when you are not feeling so great or when you are tempted to veer off your path. The letter should contain a complete description of your ideal life and what it would look like if your greatest dreams were achieved. Place this letter in a safe place so that you can remember to read and refer to it when needed.

A *Vision Statement* can be written at the conclusion of the year for the year ahead or at any time you feel that you need to make a fresh start in life.

Begin with statements like, *"I'm worthy of…"* or *"I am…"* and conclude with inspiring ideas such as, *"It is my aim to use every ounce of my great potential in all areas of my life."* I prefer to write my Vision Statement as if it were a story. I begin it by saying, *"About this year, all I can say is, 'Wow.' I have accomplished more than I can imagine… I have achieved…"*

An example Vision Statement could read, *"I am in an excellent shape, healthy and well-toned. I work out at least forty minutes every day and have a healthy and nourishing diet. Each* *day, I work on building my skills in business and wellbeing. I now earn $XXX per month and contribute to the community. I have an excellent schedule that allows me to achieve my potential and what is important in each moment of time."*

Exercise

Write a 1-page Vision Statement of your ideal lifestyle for the new year. On New Year's Eve, have your Vision Statement printed out and placed in a protective cover. Hold this statement tightly as you step into the new year at midnight and then review it daily. This is symbolic of your commitment to hold your dream and your vision at the top of your mind as you move throughout the year.

PURPOSE AND CODE OF CONDUCT STATEMENT

It is important to recognise what your purpose is in life, and how to go about achieving it. This is what gives life true meaning. A *Purpose and Code of Conduct Statement* is about the steps you will take to realise your purpose.

Here is my Purpose and Code of Conduct Statement:

My purpose is to inspire through inspirational wisdom and through books and workshops and to help facilitate healing of body and mind with teachings of tai chi and qigong.

I am disciplined and well balanced in mind, body and spirit.

I am on schedule to being financially abundant.

No more excuses: I do my best always to achieve my highest potential in health, career and relationships and in emotional and spiritual wellbeing.

In being the best I can be to achieve my highest dreams and being resourceful, I inspire others that it's also possible for them to achieve their dreams.

Exercise

In your journal, write your own Purpose and Code of Conduct Statement.

MIND MAP

Much like aiming for the bullseye on a dartboard, a *Mind Map* helps you focus your energy on hitting your target and keeping your main objectives in sight. A Mind Map provides a clear visual overview of your priorities, offering a tailored snapshot of what's most important for you to take action on. Having a one-page visual summary of your goals in all the major areas of life can be incredibly valuable.

To recap:

- Your Vision Statement is an overview (in story form) of your ideal life for the upcoming year.

- Your Purpose and Code of Conduct Statement helps define your purpose, which can stay unchanged for many years. It is like your compass in the journey of life, helping to guide your choices and decisions.

- A Mind Map can include some elements of the above, but its essential role is as a visual summary of the current goals you are working on, with a timeframe you would like the goals to be achieved by. A Mind Map may display your goals for one year or up to three years.

Exercise

Copy the image below onto a piece of paper. You may add additional categories if they are important to you. Next, fill out the Mind Map by writing an affirmation of what you're aiming to achieve in each area of your life. An affirmation is a statement of how you would like things to be, written in the present tense as if it is already realised.

For example, next to "Spirituality" you could write, "*I have a great internal reservoir of peace, clarity, strength and wisdom gained through my daily practices of meditation, prayer, reading and listening to inspired teachings. I am aligned with my highest values and what is truly important.*"

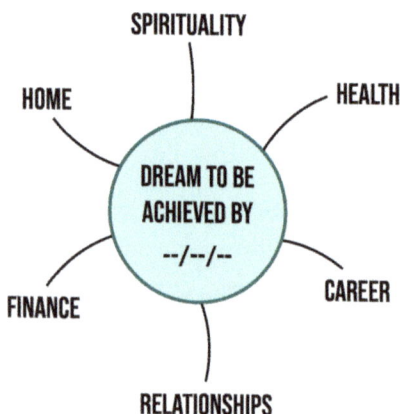

AVOID OVERWHELM

If you think about everything you have to do to reach your goals, it can be easy to feel overwhelmed. A technique I've found to prevent overwhelm is to focus on the outcome desired, then to create a plan and a list and focus on completing one step at a time. This makes it easier to accomplish what you are setting out to achieve.

Once you put together a list of all that needs to be done, it is best to then separate out those tasks in a timed schedule, giving each task a half-hour or a forty-minute segment.

The fun part of this exercise is that, after completing each task, you can tick it off or cross it out on your sheet of paper. This brings a great sense of satisfaction and helps you to visualise the progress you're making. At the conclusion of each day, it is encouraging to see the progress made and how much you accomplished.

Exercise

Pick an area of life that you feel a bit of overwhelm in. It may be because you feel there is too much to do. Write your outcome or goal if it were achieved according to your highest vision.

Make a general to-do list that lists all the steps you think may be required to reach the outcome and highlight the steps that stand out that will help you make the most progress.

Decide on a timeframe you will stick to that will assist you to accomplish your to-do list. For example, forty minutes per task. On a blank piece of paper, write in your first highlighted step or task to accomplish. For example, "*9am–9.40am: I will study best practices to achieve business goals by reading from a book by someone accomplished in this field of interest."*

Write in your next timeframe with the next action step from the list. For example, *"10am–10.40am: Action new marketing ideas."*

ACHIEVEMENTS

I believe it is of vital importance to remember all your achievements, even the little ones. If our life moves in the direction of what we focus on, then focusing on achievements will build success over the long term.

Don't discount how far you have come. Remember and be grateful for all your achievements.

At the conclusion of each year, a useful exercise is to type up all your achievements for the year and place a printed copy in a folder. This list is very useful to review in challenging times.

Another great practice for reflection is to write your daily achievements in a journal each evening. This makes it easier to recall your best achievements at the end of the year. It also helps you build momentum, encouraging your continued success and inspiring you to keep on achieving great things.

Exercise

Define your greatest achievements so far by reflecting on the past year of your life and making a list of all the great things you have accomplished.

Then, write down what you have achieved today.

CHAPTER 4

ACTION

Goals and plans into action: this is where the rubber hits the road.

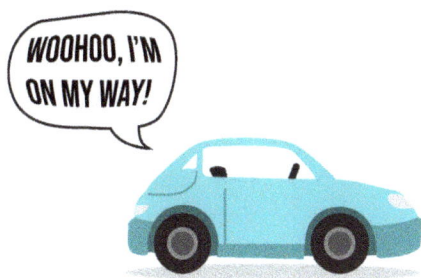

What's the point to life?
It is to truly live,
not to sit on the sidelines,
but to take a chance and do one's absolute best
in living the dream envisioned.
Believe it's possible and live it!

STEP BY STEP TO DREAM ACHIEVEMENT

There is only so long you can wish,
dream and hope.
One day, all excuses for non-action and
procrastination need to be put aside.
Little steps—they need not be grand—
can then be taken.
Achieve what they said couldn't be done, amaze
people around you but most importantly, amaze
yourself with what can be accomplished.
When you hold on to your dream and highest
vision for your life, never letting go, this is more
valuable than gold, diamonds or money.
With quiet confidence, take a step towards your
dream achievement.

When I sold my home of many years in Western Sydney and moved to the North Shore, I began a new chapter. I enrolled in a share market course, developed a habit of listening to motivational teachings from YouTube and podcasts each morning and dedicated time to reading inspiring books. I started investing in myself daily.

One day, the light bulb of belief switched on. I started to believe it was possible, that I could replace my income from working in a job, which was adequate but not my true calling, with income from share trading and teaching qigong, tai chi and an online course. Over time, this new belief helped me to take the required action steps to bring this dream to life.

Only by taking the inspired action steps each day,
bit by bit and step by step, will you bring to life
your most cherished and valued dreams.

It is very important to set aside at least one full day a week to start taking action on your greatest dreams and vision. Make sure you look at your current schedule and see if this is possible for you.

There is no harm in trying new endeavours if they are in alignment with your greatest dreams. It has been said that our biggest regrets arise from what we haven't done rather than from what we have done. Do you want your life to be a sad story of what could have been, or will you take some action now to achieve your highest dreams? Bit by bit, step by step, you can make it.

If you want to be something, be it. Take some action towards your highest goals. You cannot hope, dream, wish and pray for something consistently and then take little or no action towards its achievement. Something has got to give. You must take a chance on your dream, otherwise what is the point?

Life is so precious; time is so precious.

You cannot waste time. Take a chance and take a step towards your dream achievement.

Exercise

1. Act as if…

Just for one day, suspend disbelief. Believe it's possible that your highest dream has a chance of coming true. Step into the person you would become if you were highly confident and competent and had all the necessary qualities to bring about your dream life. Over time, the belief muscles will get stronger, and opportunities will make themselves known to help you move closer to your dream.

2. Act in alignment.

Consider the next action on your to-do list and ask, *"Is this action in alignment with what I am working towards becoming and my highest aspirations, or is some adjustment required?"* This question can help you evaluate whether your actions are essential for progressing towards your dreams or merely distractions. When asked consistently throughout the day, it can guide you towards the best path, keeping you focused and moving closer to achieving your goals.

Close your eyes for one minute and then write in your journal what you feel would be the next, most inspired action step to help you to move towards turning your dream into reality or at least to take a step in the right direction, even if the step is not an easy one.

REMEMBER YOUR WHY

It is important to remember the powerful reasons why you are taking action towards your dream. One of my personal whys for pursuing my dream is that, when I reach ninety years old and I am reflecting on my life and what I have achieved, I want to be able to say with certainty to God and to my family, "*I have accomplished what I set out to do. I have done my utmost to bring inspirational healing and wisdom to the world, and I will continue to do this for as long as I live.*"

Knowing the compelling reasons why you need to achieve your goal and dream is the fuel that will help you manifest your dream into reality.

> *When you are aligned with your purpose and functioning from a place of authenticity, you are at your most powerful.*

You need to have a powerful reason that will propel you towards living your ideal life, especially if what you have been doing is currently not working. Strength comes from belief that affirms how you would like things to be. With this strength, you can push through and transform negativity into a more empowering state of mind. When was the last time you pushed yourself to rise higher?

Exercise

1. Move away from pain.

Moving away from pain can be a powerful motivator. For example, imagine yourself at ninety years old saying, *"The reason I'm not successful is because I didn't really try. I had great ideas and potential, but I settled for a life of mediocrity, and I worked at a job I didn't really enjoy. I didn't push myself to achieve excellence."* To me, the thought of expressing that sentiment is very upsetting, and I must work diligently to ensure that doesn't happen.

Ask yourself the hard question, *"What is the cost of not following through with my highest skills, potential and purpose?"* Write down your reflections in your journal.

Next, state an affirmation of your purpose. For example:

- *"I have done my utmost to make a difference and to fulfill my potential."*

- *"I am intentional about each day. I carefully plan the night before about how I can achieve the most with my gifts, strengths and purpose, and honour God in the process."*

2. Question for the start of the day.

At the start of each day, ask, *"How would my day look if it were an outstanding day? What would I achieve, do and be?"* Although it is important to check your schedule for what needs to be done on each particular day, make sure you also place in your schedule pockets of joy.

For example, you could include a 1-hour to visit your favourite park by the water to simply enjoy the sunshine and be out in nature, which could, in turn, help you get the energy and clarity you need to tackle the harder tasks on your to-do list.

Create a list in your journal of your favourite activities—these can serve as your "pockets of joy". Then, incorporate some of them into your schedule in a way that complements, rather than interferes with, your main priorities.

DARE TO DREAM: OVERCOMING THE COMFORT ZONE

Walk in congruence with who you wish to be,
rather than settling for the comforts of the moment.
Let your desire for a better way of living be all the
encouragement you need.

There comes a time in life when staying in a comfort zone is no longer satisfying and stepping out in pursuit of a dream with all the courage you can gather becomes the best way forward. When your old way of living loses its meaning, it no longer has the power to hold you back from your destiny.

Know what you value in life and what you aspire to be, and take little steps towards this every day. Then, one day, you will wake up and find that what you once held in your heart and mind as only a dream has in fact become a reality.

When I reflect on my life, the least productive times where I did not get much accomplished were when I was just coasting along, being comfortable, not pushing myself. I am happiest when I take on challenges that allow me to strive towards something great, that build on my skill set and that help me become stronger.

For example, for many years, I was just content to work out at home with my four-kilogram dumbbell. However, when I decided to join a gym with more resources to help extend my fitness potential, I discovered that that I could pull weights of over twenty-three kilograms. My personal trainer stated, "You are stronger than you think." That little four-kilogram weight I had at home had not been helping me to reach my physical potential.

Exercise

Close your eyes for a moment and question if there are any areas of life where you're living in a comfort zone. Then, ask yourself, *"What is it I value? How can I align my life and schedule to be more in congruence with what I value?"*

Finally, ask yourself, *"What is one new action step I can take today to move out of my comfort zone and closer to my dream lifestyle?"*

THE PROMISE

Keep the agreements and promises you make to yourself so that you can see your great dream come true.

How can you see your greatest dreams realised if you do not first keep the small agreements and commitments you have made to yourself? Being disciplined with these small habits will develop a strong foundation of confidence for you to start achieving great things beyond what you thought was possible.

For example, if you set your alarm to wake you at a specific time and you just switch it off and go back to sleep, you're essentially saying, "My comfort is more important to me than following through on my plans." I know that it is sometimes difficult to get out of a warm, cosy bed, especially when it is still dark outside, but how can dreams be achieved if we always give in to what is easy and comfortable?

When you make a promise to yourself—a strong declaration and commitment to a new and better way of living—and keep it, something amazing starts to happen. Past limitations and fears start losing their grip where they were holding you back, and you can start taking inspired action to bring you closer and closer to living your best life. You start accessing hidden potentials, bringing to light gifts and abilities you never knew could be developed to such an extent, and becoming more than you could have ever imagined.

In these moments, you realise that great dreams are now becoming a reality and a way of life and making a great difference in the world, now and for years to come. It all begins with keeping the promises you make to yourself. Maintain your belief that the dream is in the process of coming true, even if it takes longer than expected. Keep the faith and take inspired action.

When I keep the commitments and promises I make in my schedule, I feel a great sense of accomplishment and satisfaction. Even if I don't get everything on my goal list done that day, as long as I have accomplished the most important tasks that will make the greatest difference in my life or the lives of others, and I feel like I am utilising my potential, I feel great happiness.

Exercise

1. New promises.

Consider which new promises and commitments you could make to help you start living your dream life.

Some examples you may like to incorporate into your daily routine are:

- 10 minutes of meditation—this will assist you with gaining clarity for the day and awareness of what is important.
- 10 minutes of reviewing your Vision Statement and most important goals.
- 30 minutes of exercise—for greater health and wellbeing.
- 20 minutes of study—for increasing knowledge in the area you wish to improve.

2. A letter to your greatest dream.

Recite the following:

> *To my greatest dream and highest potential, I am so sorry I have left you on the shelf collecting dust for so many years. I feel it's time now that I acknowledge you. Get ready, for I am shaking off the dust of procrastination, mediocrity and unfulfillment, and today is the day you emerge into the light. I am honouring you by*

*taking action steps each day that are in alignment with
my purpose, mission and values. The fear that has been
holding you back is now released, as I take a step in
courage and faith to realise my inspired destiny.*

THE FENCE-SITTER

*Believe in yourself and in your dream,
even when no-one else does.
How can you fully live your life if you do not give
everything in pursuit of your dream?*

*Fence-sitters rarely achieve much.
Don't be one.
Take a chance.
Take action.
You may one day wake up amazed at
how far you have come
towards living the life of your greatest dreams.*

We were not made to be fence-sitters in life but to recognise
the gifts within and to develop and work on them to serve
God and the world. Are you prepared to pursue your great
dreams and do whatever it takes to achieve them, or will you
put them on the backburner, hoping that someday you'll find
the opportunity to get around to them?

Dreams don't take shape by themselves. If you want to
achieve them, you need serious planning and action. You will

accomplish what you set out to achieve. It may not always be in a straightforward course, but you will arrive at the place where dreams meet reality if you stay consistent in taking inspired action in alignment with your highest vision.

VISION

Have a great vision with a belief it can come true,
plan the milestone steps,
take action on the first and next steps,
refining skills along the way.

You can run on the treadmill of life, but, unless you have a vision of why you are busy and a plan to follow and stick to (amending if necessary), the busy activities can become futile, yielding little result.

For example, having a share market trading plan that you only stick to some of the time will lead to poor results in trading. I know this from experience. You need to make a commitment to yourself, have a plan of action and then implement the plan, so you can determine if it is producing good results or not. Then, the plan can be reviewed and changed if necessary for improvements.

It is important not to just follow the path of least resistance, doing what's easiest in each moment. Visualise what it is you truly want. Plan and take action in alignment with what you truly want.

More effort is required at the beginning of any endeavour. A rocket launcher uses an incredible amount of energy to send the rocket off. But then, once it gains momentum, less

energy is required. Consider the last time you achieved success in an endeavour. Was it easy at the start, or did it require
a lot of effort and concentration? Similar to the rocket ship,
if we would like great success in a particular area, we may
need to ramp up our efforts, especially at the beginning until
momentum is achieved.

Exercise

Consider your dream and the steps that are required to get
it off the ground and for you to start being successful. Read
through your Vision Statement from the earlier section of the
book and plan out the action steps required for this month.

You may wish to draw up a yearly plan for what you hope
to achieve in each month. For example, if you want to start a
new business, in January you might draw up a business plan,
then in February you could study the best marketing and sales
techniques, and in March you could start to implement your
plan and take it from there.

WHAT IS MY NEXT STEP?

*Step into the way of living and being you always
wished you could live and be.
In other words, live your truth.
Trust and take that big step.*

I once asked a successful property investor if he had for-
mulated his goals for the year. He replied that he had some
long-term goals, but what he usually focused on was his

next step. He studied and researched what he would like to achieve next.

I believe focus happens when we are most in the present moment. Rather than stressing about how to achieve the big outcome of one's ultimate lifestyle or dream, just ask yourself, *"What is my next step?"* Then bring your full attention to achieving that next step.

Do you know all the steps to achieve your dream life at the start of your journey? Of course not. Achieving success in life involves a gradual development and refinement of one's skills and abilities, learning along the way how to get better and better.

While, at times, the way may be clear, at other times, it may not be. You may then seek guidance from within, from those who have walked the path before or from the divine through prayer and contemplation.

We may not know all the steps that will lead to dream fulfilment at the start, but what we usually do know, or can gain awareness of, is the next step. Success is not just about arriving at the place where your dreams have become a reality, it's about the journey and truly enjoying each step.

Exercise

With eyes closed and a pen and paper handy, visualise your most important dream as if it were already a reality, and then ask yourself, *"What is my most important next step?"* Write this down and take action on it.

For example, you might visualise buying your dream house. The most important next step would be to work out a way to build savings and income to move forward with this dream. What kind of deposit would you need to have, and what is one actionable step you can take this month to start the process?

FAITH

Faith means to trust that things will work out. It is so important as a prelude to taking action. Without faith that the actions will lead to great results, it can be difficult to generate motivation.

To really have faith, you must let go of all limiting beliefs and develop a new belief that your dream is possible. When you truly believe you are worthy of the dream and have faith, the steps you need to take to achieve it will become clearer.

There is a time and place where dreams come true. Stay in faith.

Faith is the opposite of fear. It is the starting ground for all great miracles. I have found the following mantra to be useful whenever I feel discouraged or tempted away from my best path: *"Be true. Stay in faith."* There is power in simple affirmations.

Whenever I feel any negative emotions creeping up, I check my faith levels and ask, *"Am I believing this situation will improve? Am I staying in faith?"* Having faith that better times are on the way encourages positive expectancy, which in turn helps good things actually come to fruition.

Be true to your highest potential and to the best of who you truly are and can be.

Exercise

Close your eyes and check in with your level of faith and hope. Can you see yourself living your dream? State firmly, "*I have trust and faith that everything will work out well and for the highest good of myself and others.*"

IMPROVE YOUR FINANCES

If abundance is gained before awareness, inner strength and wisdom, how can it be sustained? Always work on the development of wisdom and awareness.

Pull in the reins of spending. If you are happy with where you are in life and where you are financially, enjoyment comes more easily. But if you are not happy, it may be time to pull in the reins of your finances and quit buying things that don't add value to your life.

Are you on schedule with your goals? If not, maybe it is time to determine how to get ahead. For example, can you prepare more meals from home? What would happen to your budget if you allocated a smaller amount to takeaway and saved the rest? It may help you to build up the resources for longer-term goals, such as a portfolio of shares or a property purchase.

Unless you live in a rural area, where it would be difficult to get to the shops, it is useful to plan your menu only three to four days in advance. This way, there will be less wastage of food, and you are more likely to stick to your budget. When I was shopping once a week, I found I was throwing out food at the end of the week, such as fruit and vegetables. By planning only a few days in advance, you can use up what is in the pantry and fridge and only buy what is necessary.

While reducing expenditure can improve abundance, bear in mind that spending time in inspiring places can put us in the right energetic space to then inspire ideas on how to generate greater abundance. So it is important to also save up for such places and experiences and savour them.

I believe that, rather than asking the question, *"How can I become rich?"*, you should ask yourself the better question, *"How can I ensure I'm doing everything possible to earn more, save more and invest wisely?"*

Develop more than one stream of income

Striving for *Multiple Sources of Income* (MSI) is a great idea, because, if one income source dries up, others can step in to fill the gap. Once MSI are established, it also provides you with greater freedom of choice over your career, allowing you to let go of roles or responsibilities that no longer bring you joy.

A finance expert once said that relying on a single source of income is not financially responsible. This resonates in today's world where job security is increasingly uncertain. Fortunately, there are countless resources available to help you generate additional income streams, including books, podcasts, YouTube channels and workshops. Take the time to listen to a financial expert whose approach aligns with yours and learn from their wisdom.

Begin by assessing your current skills. Is there something you're already good at or enjoy that could become an income-producing venture? For instance, if you're an accomplished musician, you could begin tutoring others. If you enjoy looking after animals, you might offer dog-walking or pet-sitting services for people in your area.

MSI can come in various ways, such as investment income through dividends from shares, business income from a chosen side hustle or royalty income from writing books or other creative pursuits. By diversifying your income streams, you not only increase your financial stability but also open the door to greater freedom and opportunities.

STATE MANAGEMENT

First, tell yourself, "I can make it," and then take the action steps to make it.
Keep up the momentum and keep working on an inspired vision to actualise your true potential.

State management is having the ability to recognise if you are in an empowered state or a non-inspired state and being able to adjust depending on what you are aiming to achieve.

If you're about to start work for the day, it's beneficial to begin with your shoulders back, your breathing relaxed, a clean desk and an organised to-do list. These small preparations can help you enter an optimal state for productivity and focus. Conversely, if you're winding down for sleep at the end of the day, a calm, relaxed and slower state of being is ideal. Each state of being serves its purpose, and aligning your mindset with the task or time of day can make all the difference.

Check in with yourself at various points throughout the day. Check in by asking yourself these questions: "*What state am I in? Is it an inspired or uninspired state?*" If you are in an uninspired state, ask, "*What can I do to improve?*" Ideas include improving your posture, breathwork, exercising, practising gratitude and remembering your dream.

What would happen if you threw everything at your dream? Instead of tiptoeing around, what if you worked out your next step and gave it everything you have?

If you have ever attempted to walk over burning coals with bare feet (in a carefully supervised situation!), you would have learned that you need to move into a powerful state. You check your posture is correct, clench both fists and state, "I can do this." You then gaze at the other side of the burning coals and walk across them with confident determination.

The same process can be applied to your dream:

1. Know your dream (the destination).
2. Move into positive vibration (for example, by having excellent posture, using deep breathing techniques and stating a positive affirmation).
3. Step with purpose, each day, to move closer to what you're aiming for.
4. Keep moving until you reach the destination.

AFFIRMATION FOR TAKING ACTION

Review your personal affirmations often, particularly in challenging times. This helps keep you on the same wavelength as your vision and goals.

Here is one of my affirmations. You can use this one or write one that is meaningful to you.

> I am a quiet achiever: slowly but steadily I take action towards the achievement of my most cherished dreams. I may not always feel like taking action, but I know all the effort and the overcoming of any challenges I face will be worth it when I begin to see my dream starting to be realised.
>
> To live and take action in accordance with my highest dream and vision for life is to live successfully. To not give it my all—the development and refinement of my gifts—would be to waste the precious resource of time and delay my dream achievement.
>
> I have something of great value to offer the world, and I will take action now.

OVERCOME DISTRACTIONS

*It is important to stop being distracted
from your mission.
You know what it is that you're here to do,
so set up a plan and begin action at once.*

I have observed that, in today's society, many people are addicted to their phones. Every notification ping can distract them and disrupt their focus. Because of this, I keep my phone at a distance when I'm working and studying.

I have found that, unless my day is carefully planned and I am using a time-conscious schedule aligned with my personal and business goals of the day, it is very easy to fall into procrastination or laziness. Relaxation on a scheduled day of rest is perfectly fine, but the other six days of the week require good scheduling for things of importance to be accomplished and for satisfaction to be experienced at the end of each day. Making progress and steady improvement can help generate joy and satisfaction.

It may be beneficial to avoid looking at your phone for the first hour of the morning. You could also consider assessing the notifications on your phone. Research shows that each time your phone makes a noise, it can take several minutes to refocus on the task at hand.

Keep a timetable of what needs to be done in each hour of the day (except when you are on holiday or resting), as this can keep you on track. It is also useful to carry with you your most important goal to review often and remind you of what you're working towards.

If you find yourself becoming distracted, ask yourself, "*Do I need a change in environment, such as a short walk outside, to help me refocus on the tasks at hand?*"

Exercise

Evaluate how many times a day you are distracted. Keeping a time log of where your time is being spent can be a great way to develop greater awareness, especially if things need to change. Start keeping a notebook on hand and write down a time and activity log. Alternatively, you may have a diary that has hourly time divisions marked. Write in how you are spending your time.

What can you do to ensure there are quality scheduled times to focus?

BIG STEP

You can take little steps, one by one, to be better than yesterday. Then, one day, life may call on you to take a big step, a leap over, to land in your new way of life so you can take a big chance on your dream. These transformational opportunities need to be acted on if they align with your highest values and vision.

> *Don't be too scared to take a big step, if you feel in your heart and spirit that a big step is needed.*

One morning, about two years ago, I felt in my spirit that my role in administration was no longer right for my career and I needed to let it go to pursue my dreams. This was a big step, as I had not developed much in the way of alternative income. But I took the step anyway, and I began to draw on my other skills. I started utilising my twenty years of experience in practising tai chi to teach classes, and I also increased my study of share trading and subsequently my trading improved. Bit by bit, my income levels started to show improvement.

Exercise

Ask yourself, *"What lessons do I need to learn from what life is showing me now? Do I need to be more assertive and confident? Is there a big step I need to take a chance and action?"*

In those moments, you need to avoid uncertainty, as it wastes a lot of energy. If you know you can do something, why not do it and take a chance?

PERSONAL GROWTH

If you immerse yourself in the education and experience of personal growth by listening to motivational messages, reading inspiring books, practising visualisation and affirmations, making plans and taking daily action steps towards your ideal lifestyle, you will elevate your life and unlock your full potential to achieve all you were meant to be.

It's all about scheduling. Are you making time in your schedule for these good, productive habits? Instead of listening to music while getting ready for the day, I have made it a habit to listen to educational podcasts on personal growth and finance from select mentors I admire and wish to learn from. This one practice alone has helped me immensely in keeping a positive attitude and in developing new skills and learnings that can enhance my life. It also makes for interesting conversations with others, as you can share your learnings.

I believe that, if you are diligent in working on your gifts every day, you will make breakthroughs and miracles will occur. You will greatly impact the lives of others and make a difference in the world. You never know how far your reach will be when you diligently aim to improve each day.

For example, I am diligent with my writing after meditation practice each day. Even if I write only one impactful sentence in my journal, I feel I am progressing my skills. One sentence may not seem like much; however, I am aware that, sometimes, it only takes one powerful sentence to bring about transformation in someone's life. I have listened to many powerful, amazing speakers, and often it is just one sentence they say that completely resonates with me, changes how I view things and helps me to propel forward.

Exercise

Think about a great teacher or mentor you would like to learn from. Can you incorporate more time to learn from them into your schedule. Can you listen to their podcast while you get ready for the day or allocate time to read their books?

Evaluate and write in your journal what skills you have and what you would like to work on. How can you apply diligence to improve those skills? For example, if you feel you have skills and talent in a particular sport and would like to improve, is there a great mentor you could contact who might be open to training you?

COMMITMENT

The ultimate skill that will allow you to achieve your dream is unwavering commitment.

Back when I was training in karate, I attended a tournament where the head of the club, alongside his instructors, gave some demonstrations on the power of commitment. I watched in awe as the head instructor yelled a loud, "Kiai!"

and broke twenty-five roof tiles in a single, swift downward punch. Then, I watched in amazement as my instructor broke a piece of wood suspended in mid-air. These powerful performances showed that a singular focus on the outcome, with no hesitation, leads naturally to achieving one's goals.

Commitment is action without hesitation.

Ask yourself, *"Do I want this goal or not?"* Dabbling is not going to produce your desired results. Release anything holding you back. Your dream needs to be clear and compelling enough to overcome all excuses for inaction and procrastination, with a supportive plan to help you to achieve that dream.

If you do the work; say the affirmations; visualise the dream achieved; and take the action steps every day to assist with bringing the dream to life with total commitment, persisting and not backing down until the dream is realised, life and the universe may give you what you seek. But the best reward will be what you become as a result of having a dream and striving towards its achievement.

When you have something great to work towards and don't give up on it, something remarkable happens: you develop your inner strength and resolve, strengthen your character and become a better person. Are you giving it your all to be successful? If not, you may like to state the following:

> I have had enough of not trying, not being successful, not giving it my all. I'm placing those days behind me. It's time for a change. What if, for the

next month, I give my dreams everything I have? I will determine what my highest goals and priorities are and just go for it.

Feel the strength within. You have what it takes to achieve this great dream.
Believe and achieve.

Exercise

Evaluate your present goals and determine if you are giving them total commitment by allocating proper time towards them each day.

If you find you are not making commitment towards your goals, revisit Chapter 1 and determine if this goal or dream is one you really would like to see come true. If you discover it's not, then start the process of visualising and dreaming all over again.

DISCIPLINE

When my family and friends see my commitment to waking up early, exercising daily and eating healthy meals on a regular basis, they often say, "You are so disciplined." To me, it's about having big goals and dreams that I would like to come true, and I view discipline and implementation of excellent habits as the path to making them a reality.

The easy road is not necessarily the best road if you would like to achieve something great with your life. The easy road often means doing the bare minimum to get by.

The harder, more challenging road involves the application of discipline. Discipline to get up early. Discipline to follow a morning routine such as meditating, exercising and reading. Discipline in mindset, with a no-excuse mentality for taking action on your dreams.

It would be easy to give in all the time to what you want to do in the moment—to do what is enjoyable and fulfilling momentarily, like eating junk food, watching too much TV, listening to uninspiring music, giving too much attention to social media or staying in your comfort zone without stiving for improvement—but at what cost? A lazy person just hoping things will get better may be bitterly disappointed.

Knowing what not to do is as important as knowing what to do.

Life, like time, is so precious—our most valuable resource. If we squander time, it does not come back. Bit by bit, the lack of a disciplined plan and action can erode your self-confidence, time, self-esteem and self-respect. But the opposite is also true: discipline builds your dream life. It's so important to take time for quiet meditation and walks along the coast; to eat healthy, nourishing foods; and to take meaningful, purposeful action on your dream life.

Discipline and adherence to routine and being your best—not just for yourself but for the many lives you can contribute to and make a difference in—is important. We must remind ourselves often of the reasons behind our discipline, as this will help us to continue to take inspired action.

When there is a hesitancy in the spirit, an uneasiness of feeling, take note and don't charge forward just because, for example, you want to make someone else happy. Your destiny and future success are worth more than this.

Self-discipline means doing what is not easy in scheduled times. This can help generate more time to re-energise and more time to accomplish what you are really here to accomplish. A life that is carefully planned and scheduled, while also allowing for rest time and at least one day a week to rejuvenate, produces more chance of freedom and accomplishment than a mentality of getting by and putting off action until a later time.

> *Disciplined action and being true to your*
> *dream and highest vision for life are*
> *what produce the results of the dream life*
> *that you wish for.*

Without discipline, virtue can be thrown out the window. Dreams, visions and plans for the future must be placed on hold. How can you accomplish anything without courage and discipline? How can you move closer to achieving a dream if you're giving all your time to the comfort zone? You must want the dream more than you want to sink back into familiar habits and do what is comfortable.

Is your dream worth fighting for? Is your dream worth giving up the love of leisure and laziness? Until it is, you don't really have a strong enough dream.

Work on finding a dream worthy of your time, efforts and commitment like your life depends on it—because it does.

HOW MUCH WOULD YOU LIKE YOUR DREAM TO COME TRUE?

I've discovered that whenever I feel discouraged or unmotivated, the key to getting back on track is to reassess how much I truly want to achieve my dream.

A great dream will help to create the inspired action steps to achieve it.

One year, I didn't reach the income goal I had set for myself. Instead of sinking into discouragement, I took the time to evaluate why this goal still mattered to me, identify areas for improvement and outline new steps to take moving forward. This process renewed my focus and gave me a clearer path ahead.

I also realised that if everything had gone perfectly according to plan, I might have fallen into complacency. Challenges and disappointments, while difficult, can serve as powerful motivators, transforming into the fuel needed for improvement. They push us to seek better strategies, uncover hidden talents and tap into our full potential.

How much do you want your dream to come true? Ask yourself this whenever you feel tempted to stray from your path. In those moments of temptation, reflect: do you want this dream more than the temporary comfort of a packet of chips or the ease of the TV remote? If your goal is to achieve your ideal body and health, choose actions that align with that vision—reach for your running shoes, your exercise bike or a nourishing juice. Each choice you make brings you closer to the life you truly want.

In each moment, you have the power of choice. You have the power to take action that aligns with your dream and highest vision instead of doing what is easier in the moment. At times, you can rest to regain energy and resolve, but don't give up or quit on the little things you could do today to move closer to living your ideal lifestyle or dream. Over time, little actions can add up, just like money that is saved over time, to build something substantial.

How strongly would you like your dream to come true? How much you would really like your dream life to move into reality is proportionate to the amount of planning and action you take. If you find yourself reverting into past habits of non-action, rejuvenate your energy by doing things like taking a walk in the park and asking yourself, *"How much would I really like this great dream to come true?"*

Exercise

If you find yourself sinking back into comfortable, non-supportive habits, have these questions on hand:

- *Is my dream worth it, or should I just go back into doing what is comfortable and easy?*
- *How can I incorporate greater discipline into my life?*

- *What new disciplines do I need to implement that can help with my dream life?*
- *Do I choose daily disciplines that can propel me to success or not even try?*
- *To not try is a path that leads to nowhere. Is nowhere where I would like to be?*
- *Would I like to make something wonderful of my life and the gifts and talents God has given me?*
- *What new discipline can I implement today in my schedule?*

SUPERSIZE DREAM

If you can do something well on a small scale, determine if it can be supersized to do well on a larger scale. We are not here to play small. If you have achieved great results in an area of your life, determine if this area could be supersized into something bigger, or at the very least shared with others in the form of tuition or mentorship.

For example, if you have a skill in teaching art, could you create an online course to reach a wider audience of students?

Exercise

Reflect on the current skills and achievements you have right now and determine if you can increase your reach with them.

GIVE IT YOUR BEST

Be satisfied only with your best. Ask often, *"Am I giving my very best effort in this situation or goal?"* Half-hearted attempts rarely produce good results. Give your all to be your very best. Life tends to favour those who put in consistent effort to improve each day.

Back in my karate days, we had to bow at the door before entering the dojo. This was to symbolise letting go of any issues of the day that could interfere with training. Once inside, we dedicated ourselves to training and giving our best effort, making it a way of life.

Exercise

Ask yourself right now if you are doing your very best to be outstanding. If the answer is no, ask why. There may be some issues that require resolving.

If you find you are not giving a task your best effort, this is the perfect opportunity to review your Vision Statement and goals. It is also the time to question, *"Do I need to change my strategy? Should I seek education to improve my skills in this area?"*

MAKE YOUR HEALTH A HIGH PRIORITY

What are the consequences of neglecting your health and failing to take inspired action towards your dreams? You risk becoming trapped in a cycle of constant complaints—"This hurts," and, "That hurts." When you have the opportunity to maintain a balanced diet and challenge yourself to exercise daily, you can significantly reduce the risk of many health concerns.

I have observed this firsthand with a family member who consistently indulged in unhealthy foods such as chips, battered fish, fizzy drinks and sweets while avoiding exercise altogether. Over time, this lifestyle led to numerous health problems and illnesses. In the years leading up to their admission to a nursing home, efforts to encourage healthier habits were met with resistance. Visiting them in the nursing home was difficult, as their greatest wish was to return home—a wish that could not be fulfilled due to the high level of care they required. Most conversations I had with them during these visits centred on the pain and discomfort they were experiencing, serving as a stark reminder of the long-term consequences of neglecting health and wellbeing.

It was in those conversations that I vowed to make health maintenance a top priority in my life. Usually, our elders are there to teach us what to do, but in this instance I learned what not to do. Never underestimate the importance of good nutrition and regular exercise—they are the foundation of good health and wellbeing.

Ask yourself, *"Where is health maintenance on my schedule, and is it given a high priority?"* For example, are you allocating at least half an hour a day to exercise? You may wish to exercise in the early morning so that it's done before you start work and so you won't get distracted by other important activities or tasks.

Physical exercise for dream achievement

Strong in motion.
Strong in spirit.

Powerful actions generate strength of spirit. This strength can then help give you the energy required to nourish your most cherished dreams and wishes into reality.

What I love about tai chi and qigong practice is that each beautiful, flowing, energetic movement works to bring about a gentle shift in energy, helping you to move from an uninspired state to an inspired state. The gentle nature of the movements helps to release any blockages, allowing a free flow of energy. It is also great for the improvement of circulation and balance and for developing strength in the body.

It is important to find an exercise you love to do that will build strength and resilience and bring harmony to the body and mind. Going on long walks, weightlifting, riding a bike, swimming and stretching are great activities to consider.

PLANS INTO ACTION

With renewed hope in your heart and clarity of vision for what you would like to achieve, it's time to put your plans into action. Get to work. No more daydreaming of what you plan to do—just do it.

Imagine your dreams as already achieved and start work from that state of being. Have a plan, work the plan and enjoy the journey. Be firm in following your action plan.

Remember to be proactive, because if you do nothing, you get nothing.

Don't think of completing mundane tasks that are in alignment with your highest vision as a chore. Think of them as **stepping stones** that are helping you to move closer to dream achievement. Work quietly and consistently towards your dream achievement. Your breakthrough will come.

CHAPTER 5

OVERCOMING OBSTACLES

When life knocks you down,
don't be fooled,
this is just temporary.
Soon, if you keep aiming to be your best,
you will rise and, one day, shine.

DON'T PUT YOUR DREAMS ON HOLD

Become the person you have always
dreamed you could be.
No holding back.
You are loved by God and by those you hold dear.
You can make a difference.
You do matter.

If you're in a low-energy state and you're not truly grateful for all you have now, it can be easy to put your dreams on hold. Gratitude energises and uplifts, allowing you to give your best effort towards your goals. Without it, you may find it difficult to move forward, as you cannot give what you do not have within yourself.

I understand this all too well. For many years, I was caught up in the relentless treadmill of life, working tirelessly just to make ends meet and using my spare time to keep the house in order. This didn't turn around until I started to put into practice true appreciation and began to believe my dream was possible. I listened to inspiring teachings every day, cultivated discipline, and took inspired action towards dream achievement.

Right now, you may have placed your dreams on hold, waiting and hoping for that one magical day when everything will come together to enable your dream to be realised. But what if the dream itself holds the golden ticket for its own realisation? Every time you visualise your dream life, visit the place of your dreams, believe deeply and give thanks, you bring your dream closer to being realised.

There is one thing that can be a great comfort and strength in times of misfortune, and that is a vision of a better tomorrow.

Obstacles can arise when we lose sight of who we truly are and what we're aiming for or when we start to believe that our goals are unattainable. We are spiritual beings having a human experience. Everyone has a great gift to nourish and bring to the world. If you forget who you are and what wonderful gift you can offer the world, it's very easy to run into obstacles. This is because it can affect our focus and subsequent energy generation. For example, if our focus is that, "I don't really have something great I can bring to the world," then it could result in poor outcomes. Instead, if you focus on what you can do and an area of life you have a strength in and believe, "I can improve my gifts and make a difference one day," then this belief can help generate more positive outcomes. Know what you are aiming for and keep your focus on your dream, and you will not be lost in all the details of how to get there. Stay in tune with your inner awareness to discern the right action for each moment of time.

It is not in the easy times that we develop or test our strength; it's in the challenging times. When you overcome obstacles and hurdles, it makes you stronger.

Strength of spirit can be felt when you believe, "*I can make it! If I fall, I will get up.*"

INNER PEACE

Let no-one disturb the place of inner peace within.
It helps to develop a wellspring of inner strength
in times of need.
Trust all is well and will be well.

Life, with all its demands and distractions, can often throw unexpected challenges our way. To navigate these effectively, it's crucial to carve out time each day just for yourself—time to build your foundation of resilience by connecting with the peace and calmness within.

My morning practice of prayer and meditation is a must each day. It is in these times of silence that I cultivate and reinforce my inner strength, preparing myself for any challenges the day may bring.

Think about your morning routine. Is it setting you up with the peace, calmness and strength you need?

Exercise

Make a list of what brings you peace of mind. For example, do you find that spending time in beautiful, inspiring environments helps? Or spending time in solitude, listening to the whispers of your heart and appreciating all you have?

Check your schedule and see if there is a way you can make this part of your weekly or even daily practice. Practise bringing the peace you have generated from this exercise into any challenging situations you may face, having faith and trust that all is working out for the best.

A NEW BEGINNING

Each day is a new beginning,
a new chance to be creative,
a chance to let go of what has not been working
and to start over.
A chance to make things right.

It's a new day; let it be that.
No need to drag any past remorse into today.
Let it be.

Time is valuable; this date and time will never
come again.
You have to make the most of it.

It is time to let go of regret and past mistakes and make a new start. Your visions and dreams for the future are so important. Hold on to them dearly, for they will hold you to a higher standard than you have currently been living at.

A great vision helps you to build the discipline necessary and do what it takes to achieve your dream. However, keep in mind that progress is more important than perfection. If you are making progress each day towards your vision and goals, this will lead to fulfilment and joy in life.

For example, a failed relationship does not mean that future relationships are destined to fail. By treating each day as a new beginning, you can create a renewed vision of what you are seeking in an ideal partner and outline these qualities clearly. Taking proactive steps, such as attending social events or exploring platforms for meeting like-minded individuals, can set you on the path to building meaningful connections. Each step forward brings you closer to forming fulfilling relationships and discovering new possibilities.

Evaluate in your life where you would like to start over. Treat today as a truly new day.

Exercise

Design what an outstanding day would look like for you, then an outstanding week.

An outstanding week that brings great joy and peace to your life consists of seven truly wonderful days; it could then extend to be the best year of your life so far.

For example, an outstanding day may begin: "I wake up at 5am, before the sun rises. I feel gratitude fill my heart as I get to choose what I do today. I exercise for 40 minutes, as it helps me feel wonderful and alive and keeps me in shape. I then work on what is truly important to me."

YOU ARE CLOSER THAN YOU THINK

If we think our dreams are far away and not achievable in the near future, it becomes easy to give up or even backtrack. But what if your greatest dream is just around the corner? What if it's closer than you think?

It is easy to feel depressed if you think of how far away your dream is and all the effort and resources required to realise it. The key to overcoming this is a combination of faith, vision and action. Each time you visualise your dream, believe in its potential and take disciplined steps—no matter how small—you bring yourself closer to making it a reality.

For example, when you look in the mirror and see how much work is required to reach your ideal body shape, close your eyes and visualise the version of yourself as you aspire to be. Picture yourself in beautiful, stylish clothes, your hair and face looking radiant and youthful, your body well-toned and looking better than it's ever been. Then, work out a plan, schedule it in your diary, prepare your exercise clothes and adjust your diet by researching the best and most nutritious foods and drinks. Finally, and most importantly… TAKE ACTION.

Tomorrow is going to come along whether you move in alignment with your dreams or not, but why not give your dreams a chance? You may surprise yourself when one day you wake up and are actually living the life you only dreamed about years earlier.

Gratitude, reverence for life and knowing that each day is a gift from God can help each day be wonderful. You are worthy of living the life of your greatest dreams. Are you all in for your dream?

ROCK BOTTOM

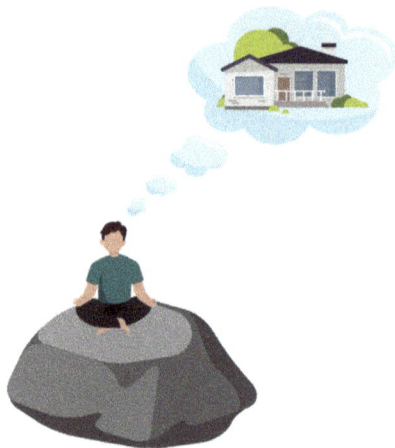

When you have hit rock bottom in life and feel great discontent, take a moment to dream and a moment to visualise this dream achieved. Feel a sense of groundedness in the resources you have now, such as your health, and speak this affirmation: *"I may not know all that is involved in achieving this dream, but, with divine help and determination and strength of spirit, achieve it I will. I have what it takes to be successful! I'm going to make it!"*

Realise that rock bottom can be the perfect time for a breakthrough. Because you cannot go any lower than this, you can start to feel the strength and stability of the rock beneath you.

Begin to visualise what you are aiming for, such as a new home, improved finances or being in your ideal career, and start to believe it is possible. Close your eyes for clarity and ask, *"What is my next step?"* Then, begin to take action at once.

My rock-bottom moment was about eight years ago. I was working full-time in a job I didn't particularly enjoy and was living in a house filled with excessive clutter. To make matters worse, my husband and I went through a separation, followed by a divorce. Determined to change my life, I began visualising and writing about what my ideal home, career and life would look like in seven years. I committed to reading that vision every day.

At first, the vision of living my ideal dream life felt hazy and distant. However, something powerful happens when you commit to reading, visualising and truly immersing yourself in the feeling of what it would be like to live your dream—and doing this consistently every day. Like a camera lens adjusting to bring a picture into focus, I discovered that the more you review and refine your dream, the sharper and clearer it becomes. As your vision comes into focus, so too do the steps you need to take to make it a reality.

My first step to improve my life was to read decluttering books. When there is order in the environment you spend a lot of time in, it helps immensely to bring order to your dreams and plans. Over the following six months, I let go of over fifty per cent of my belongings. Then, I spruced up the home and sold it. I moved to the North Shore, close to a place overlooking a beautiful harbour, with a beach only fifteen minutes away.

Spending time in beautiful environments in silence gave me the inspiration and insights I needed to make a new start in a great career aligned with my gifts and talents. It was then I requested to reduce my full-time hours at work to part time so that one day a week I could work on my ideal career.

During this time, I learned how to trade shares, began compiling my writings into a book and expanded my teachings in tai chi. After two years of living in this home with minimal belongings, I decided to pursue my dream career full time, create an online course and launch a merchandise store featuring inspirational quotes. Not long after, I moved back to my family home to assist my elderly mother, and, at the time of writing this book, I am working towards purchasing my dream home in an inspiring area.

I hope, through hearing my story, you can see that being at rock bottom is the perfect opportunity to make some great changes in life. It is a time in which a new vision for the future can be formed, and it is a great time to start over in a more inspiring direction.

Do you need to change your approach?

If you always do what you have always done, you may always achieve similar results. Do you need to make changes to your approach to dream achievement? Can you learn new skills or ideas?

One activity that has helped me immensely in learning new skills and approaches is to read a new book every week in an area I would like to excel in. Over time, I have found these new learnings, once applied, all make a big difference.

RESOURCES

Richness in life is not just about having an abundance of money. Richness is about striving for abundance in all areas, including health, relationships, emotional wellbeing, spirituality, intellectual growth and financial stability. Money is simply a resource to help you translate your plans into action.

Don't be concerned by what you do not have currently. Notice the abundance that you already have and be thankful for more abundance to appear. Excellent health, time freedom, a place to live that provides shelter from the elements, having healthy food to eat, spending time in meaningful conversations with friends and being thankful for all you have are all examples of great riches.

An artist does not see a piece of rock, ice or wood as simply that—they see what it can become. What can you make from the resources you have?

Do the best you can with the resources you have,
move past excuses,
reach for the stars
and achieve what is beyond your wildest dreams
and expectations.

The marketplace constantly tells us, "You need this. You need that," but until you find inner peace and a deep appreciation for what you already have, will acquiring more things truly make a difference?

If I had had great wealth and abundance at the beginning of my journey, would I have had the burning desire and passion to make the most of my financial resources? I don't think so. A lack of resources helps us to look more closely at what we do have and how we can become more creative if there is a dream that is strong enough to sustain us through the difficult times.

Ask yourself if, when everything is going well in life, you have the same level of motivation to be successful as you do when experiencing dissatisfaction. Vision is vitally important, but you also need the desire for improvement in some aspect of life and the will to find the solutions to bring this about.

Character is developed in tough times. You become most resourceful when facing hardships. Challenges can make you stronger and more resourceful, depending on your inner resilience.

We eventually become and achieve what we hold dearest in our hearts.
Hold on to a defeatist attitude and defeat may be yours. Hold on to hope and a vision that you have belief in, and you may see your greatest dreams become a reality.

Exercise

Consider your current resources in relation to achieving your dream. Think about all you have right now, such as good health, the ability to read and understand, the wonderful people in your life and mentors you can learn from. Consider if more resources are needed or if you can make greater use of the current ones.

Are you making use of the books you have on your shelf? Do you have access to a library? How are you reaching out to people you know who are successful in the areas you wish to be successful in? You may have more resources than you realise right now and more than you need to begin to live the life of your greatest dreams.

SADNESS

Sadness has a season,
but soon it will pass.
Like a song, there is only so long it can be played
before it becomes repetitive.
Allow the emotions of hope and positive expecta-
tion to start.
Allow this new song to play in your heart.
Soon you will see signs of spring in your life.

Sadness, despair and disgust at where you are right now in life can serve as a wake-up call that helps you to decide, *"It is no longer acceptable to live this way, be this way. I must make a change and find within my heart the song I want to sing from now on."* Remember, there are many ways to climb a mountain. What new way of living could you now dedicate your life to? Perhaps when you're on a holiday, even if for a couple of days, you can relax enough to gain a glimpse of a great vision—for example, a three-year plan for how you wish to live your newly-designed life.

Sadness is a great teacher. It can show us that we are not there yet or that we need to release or let go of something not working in our life. Do you have a dream that is tugging at your heart, saying, *"Try me, try me. Give me life. Become and achieve the highest vision that you can be and achieve"*? Sadness occurs when we ignore the dreams of the heart and carry on doing that which brings no joy.

There are gifts within that require acknowledgement to be worked on and developed. If, each day, some progress can be made towards dream achievement—even if it's just small progress—our gifts within will be developed, until one day we will live the life we once only imagined.

Let go of doubt and take a leap of faith. You are closer than you think to living the life of your greatest dreams. I feel joy much more regularly now than in years gone by, as I take daily action on following the calling of my heart and working on and utilising my gifts to serve the world. My career does not feel like work, it feels like what I was born to do.

Exercise

When you start to feel sad, ask yourself, *"What is it that I could be hopeful about? What am I looking forward to?"*

Schedule in calendar time so that you can do more of what brings joy to your heart.

MISTAKES

Mistakes

Mistakes—though they seemed as such—
I realised they taught me much.
Would I know all I do today, if I did not make
mistakes along the way?
All of us are here to learn, and through mistakes
we can discern,
different colours and sounds of the heart,
and how to become more smart,
what not to do and to do to evolve,
to reach the truth within to solve.
Mistakes—though they seemed as such—
I realised they taught me much.

We can learn a lot from mistakes. You know you are growing when you make mistakes, and you can learn what not to do or what to do better in the future.

When you realise that you have made a mistake, it is useful to reflect on the following to find clarity and resolution to avoid the mistakes being repeated:

1. What was the mistake?
2. What were the forces involved in bringing this about?
3. What can I learn from this?
4. What is the epiphany or revelation of truth from this?
5. How can I transform or reframe the above so it can help in the future?

For example, if you are in the habit of buying ready-made foods (when your goal is to become more health conscious and you can prepare your own food well), you may realise that this habit may be due to wanting food in a hurry and not being more prepared to make your own healthier options. You may need to learn to be more organised. The truth may be that you have settled for less than what is good for you because you have not taken the time to evaluate better food choices, recipes and what you can do to make food in advance. To be of better health and wellbeing, it may be worth preparing natural fresh foods from now on.

Sometimes mistakes result from not being truly connected to a higher vision for the future, thinking that dream achievement is too far away or thinking that you're not worthy of the dream. Many successful people will tell you that mistakes or failures can happen as you start to move towards your dream. Learning how to navigate around or through problems and seeing them as valuable feedback is what can build your skill set. Each challenge you overcome strengthens and equips you further, turning obstacles into opportunities for growth and development.

It is important to remember that you are valuable and you have something great to offer the world. Perhaps you have not had role models in your life demonstrating high levels of excellence. Don't let this be an excuse for not letting your true light shine. If you don't have any role models in your life in the areas in which you wish to succeed, head to the nearest bookshop and learn from the best. There are also many YouTube videos or podcasts featuring successful ideas that you can start your learning from. Then, once you find an excellent mentor, you may like to attend one of their courses or workshops.

Learning from an experienced mentor can help you avoid common mistakes by benefiting from their knowledge and experience—there's no need to reinvent the wheel. It is a wise approach to learn about the best practices and procedures in your field from successful people as well as understanding what to avoid.

For example, in the realm of share trading, I learned from my mentor that it is best to have a pre-determined stop-loss before you buy the shares; this way you will know at what point it is best to sell if the trade does not go as planned. This can help prevent the mistake of losing more in the trade than is acceptable.

Have compassion for where you are currently. There is great power in understanding and accepting where you currently stand in life and your achievements.

Rise up and be that person you were created to be.
No more living in denial of what can be.

Exercise

Ask yourself:

- *What are your mistakes teaching you now?*
- *Is there a new skill you wish to learn?*
- *Who are the role models you can learn from?*
- *What is the best way to put into practice these new skills and learnings?*

ACTUALISING POTENTIAL

Push it to the limit.
To really know what you are capable of,
push to the limit of your potential.
Give your dream everything you have.

You are capable of so much, so why settle for only using a small part of your potential? Why not give your all in the pursuit of your dreams and see what happens? At the very least, you'll have the satisfaction of knowing that you are doing and being all you can do and be in order to live your best life.

Don't just dip your toe in the water.
Dive right in.
Be committed to your highest potential and the
greatest dream you have.

It is not a pleasant feeling when you know you are only using a small part of your potential and skill set. I know this all too well, having spent fifteen years in an unfulfilling administration role, constantly feeling that I was capable of so much more.

My strongest skills, which I have thoroughly enjoyed developing, include creative and inspirational writing, teaching tai chi, exploring life-improvement concepts and applying newly learned ideas to enhance personal growth. When I finally started to acknowledge the calling from God and from within, it was time to start developing and utilising more of the skills that I am passionate about and that bring to the light the higher visions and dreams I have in my heart, so I could be of greater service to the world.

Put your gifts to work. Why hide them when it might just make a huge difference in someone's life, and your own, for the better? A friend of mine is an excellent example of fully utilising one's potential. Despite being over seventy-five and suffering from arthritis and other health conditions, she remains committed to staying active. Each morning, she wakes up before 5am and pushes herself to walk for an hour, knowing that this routine helps with her circulation, builds strength and keeps her healthy. I was amazed at how well she was walking when I last saw her. Her dedication is a testament to the power of perseverance, even in the face of physical challenges.

Exercise

Here's an exercise to help you seek direction that is in alignment with your highest vision and have the energy to achieve it.

After you reach a relaxed state through deep breathing and excellent posture, ask yourself the following questions and write down the answers:

- *What is my highest potential in health? What does it look like?*
- *What is my highest potential in relationships, both in my family and personal life?*
- *What is my highest potential in career?*
- *What is my highest potential in finances?*
- *What is my highest potential in spiritual renewal?*

You can apply the same strategy to other important areas of life to gain insights and identify opportunities for improvement.

Record your new understandings of potential in a journal and then work out the action steps you can take towards achieving your highest potential.

TOOLKIT

We usually have a toolkit in the home for when something needs to be fixed. Why not have a toolkit on hand for any time you feel tired, lazy, unmotivated or sad or when you're about to give up on your vision and goals?

Here are some examples of a toolkit that can be handy if you need to realign yourself towards your highest dream and goals:

1. **Meditate** for 10 minutes. This can act as a refreshing boost to give you a second wind, a new energy to get up and start achieving again.

2. A **walk** for 15 minutes or more in fresh air and beautiful scenery can help with clearing the mind and restoring your energy levels. Taking a walk is a great way to think through solutions to whatever is troubling your mind. You will be amazed at the wisdom that can flow through. While you're walking, remind yourself who you really are and what your gifts are and think about how you can develop them.

3. **Qigong and tai chi.** These practices will help you gain inner peace, tranquillity and renewal at deep levels. For

a recommended qigong routine, check out my online course at www.wisdomandhealingqigong.com.au.

4. **Listen** to inspirational messages on YouTube or a favourite song that uplifts the spirit.

5. **Make a healthy juice.** One of my favourites is the following recipe: half a cucumber, a handful of baby spinach and the juice of half a lemon or grapefruit blitzed with some water.

6. **Read** an inspirational book for 15–20 minutes, followed by your list of achievements, vision, goals or dreams.

7. **Declutter** for 20–40 minutes. This brings about a great sense of accomplishment and clarity of mind, as well as an understanding of what is important. It also gives you a feeling of pride when you can show the newly cleared area to others. Once you've cleared one area, you will gain the motivation to clear other areas, until the whole house is done. When you walk around the home, you will feel encouraged and at peace.

8. **Pray and affirm**. Affirmations and prayers allow you to visualise how you wish your life to be. For example, *"Thank you for the great abundance and riches flowing in my life."*

9. **Visit a place** that brings inspiration to your spirit. This could be a park, the beach, a favourite café or an excellent restaurant you have saved for. It could be a special place in the mountains where you can reflect and admire nature's great beauty.

UNEMPLOYMENT OR TIMES OF GREAT CHALLENGE

*If the present state of where you are right now
in relation to dream and finances appears bleak,
your future does not have to look bleak also.
What you may need is to develop a fighting spirit.*

Say to yourself, "*I will not let this defeat me; I have the means to work out a way through this to a time of financial abundance.*"

Identify and write down what resources you do have—resources of wisdom, health and financial assets. Keeping these in mind, create an action plan that will guide you in moving forward effectively.

Know that you have the support of the creator of this universe. Say a prayer of gratitude and thanks for what you do have. Give a seed or portion of what you have for higher purposes, such as to your church or charity of choice. And then, with an inner battle cry, start to implement your plan of action.

*You've got to fight for your dreams.
Connect to inner strength.
Have a strong spirit.
You've got this.
You can achieve this.*

JOURNEY INTO WHOLENESS

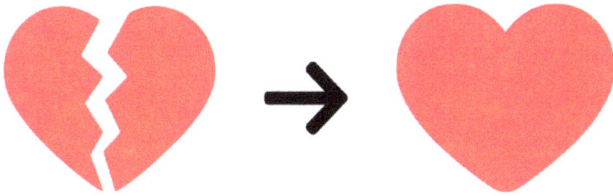

Appreciate every moment. It is a gift from God.

"Our creator is not interested in your past mistakes; he is interested in what your future can be from now on. It's not too late to fulfil your destiny and purpose." When I heard this from a minister, something stirred in my heart. The eagle's wings started to awaken.

At a success seminar where Tony Robbins was a guest speaker, I learned about the power of appreciation and how it can elevate your state of wellbeing. He discussed how to be in a beautiful state and be free from suffering. We were asked to recall three times we felt a deep appreciation for something and to then bring these experiences and memories back into the heart centre.

I recalled:

1. The birth of my daughter: seeing her for the first time and thinking what a miracle she is.

2. Returning to the moment when, as a twenty-one-year-old, I became a world champion in karate. I visualised myself sitting down at the place where I

was staying in Canada, gazing at the six-foot trophy under the window and feeling immensely grateful for that opportunity.

3. When I was driving to pick up the keys to my new home that I had carefully saved for seven years for. I was so proud.

As I felt this deep appreciation, held a strong stance and said, "Yes!", anchoring my appreciation with a tightly held fist, I felt a shift in my state. I was not yet, at the time of the seminar, what you would call "financially abundant". I had not yet achieved the vision I had for my life, but, nevertheless, this eagle lifted off the ground and started to soar. I felt a wholeness and a knowing that I have what it takes to be successful.

I started to feel with certainty that I could bring these dreams I held so dear to my heart into reality. I knew I could make it in this world. I knew I could make a difference and inspire others—not just through my words but through example.

What if the next five to twenty years are actually the best years of your life so far, and all the hardship and negative feelings or experiences of the past have actually made you who you are today: more grateful and appreciative, stronger and more resilient; with wisdom, strength of character and genuine compassion for others?

If one has everything given to them on a silver platter, they may not have the appreciation or wisdom to sustain this good fortune. Just look at the statistics of lottery winners—how many still have the great wealth, not just in money but in life experiences, three years after winning?

If life has not been easy for you up until now, consider that it's building up your inner strength, knowledge and wisdom and generating creative ways for you to bring about a wonderful, beautiful life.

Exercise

With your eyes closed for a few minutes, consider what can be. What beliefs or mistakes do you need to gently let go of to make space for the new? What can you be appreciative of right now?

REST, CALMNESS AND JOY FOR REJUVENATION

It is very important to allow yourself a day of rest once a week—a day where you can dream, reflect and recharge your batteries. This can help refresh you and keep you motivated.

For most people, weekdays are filled with many tasks. Why not allow yourself a day to just be? This is a day when you have nowhere to rush off to, no tasks that need completion. You can just rest in the moment. There is great power in restoration, in just being.

It is important to reconnect to the grounding energy of nature, such as by visiting a beautiful park, lake or beach. There is nothing like the feeling of the warm sun and a soft breeze to help you feel connection to the earth, to restore peace and harmony to body and mind. Remember, we are not machines.

We cannot be revved up all the time. One's best work, output and creativity can arrive from a state of calmness. For instance, I find that my most inspired writing happens when I'm surrounded by nature.

Value time and this moment—they are what life is made of.

If things aren't going right, take a moment to find something humorous and enjoy a good laugh. Laughter can restore your energy levels and fuel your next endeavour with renewed vitality.

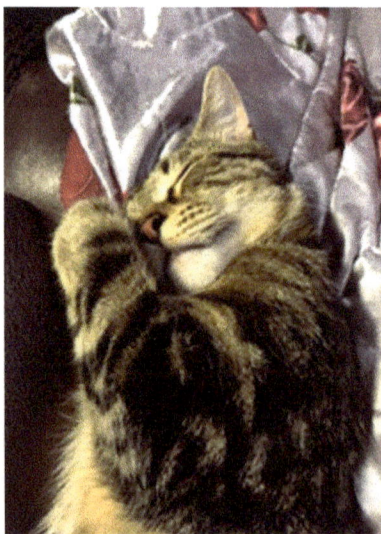

There is nothing like a pet to cheer you up. After a long, hard day at work, having your cat sleep on your lap can bring joy to the heart. The photo on the previous page is of my cat Simba when he was just a kitten. Isn't he just adorable?

Simba makes me laugh, especially when he rolls on his back in the sun or tries to hide under my quilt on a cold day. Also, whenever there is a bag or box lying around, he will jump into it. He loves bags.

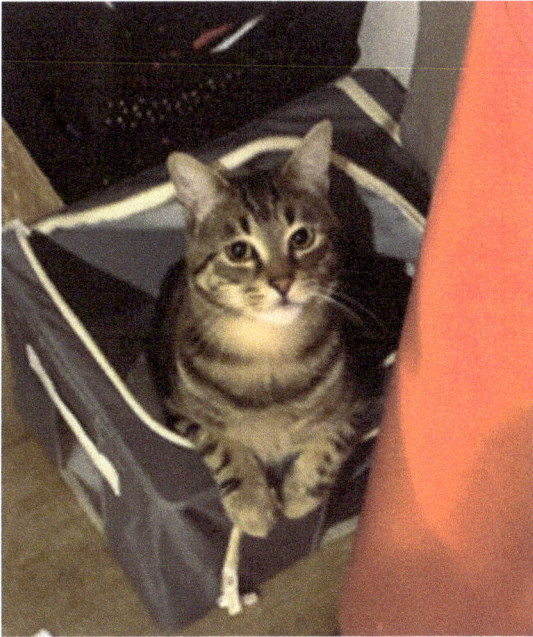

Some people enjoy watching comedy shows to bring laughter into their lives, but developing the ability to let go of excessive seriousness, relax in the moment and appreciate what brings peace and joy can be just as uplifting.

Determine what makes you laugh, whether it's spending time with uplifting people, enjoying the company of pets or listening to something funny. Take a moment now to smile and enjoy a good laugh.

Exercise

1. Check in.

Check in with yourself by asking:

- *Am I getting enough sleep?*
- *Am I allowing time for meditation?*
- *Am I eating healthy foods and limiting caffeine?*
- *Do I have a pet I can care for? Or, otherwise, a plant? A beautiful garden can also bring much joy.*

2. Little joys.

Write down a list of little joys that can help to brighten your day, and action some of them. The list may include:

- buying flowers to brighten up the house
- spending time outdoors and feeling the warmth of the sun on your body
- enjoying the first sip of your morning coffee
- exploring new areas you have not yet been to
- having a day off mundane work
- looking out to sea and feeling gratitude in the depths of your being
- looking in the mirror and stating, *"I have what it takes to be successful. I really do."*

RESPONSIBILITY

While we may not have control over what happens in life, we do have control over how we respond to what happens and the attitude we choose to adopt.

When you do well with what you have, you will be entrusted with more and more. This is a biblical principle, such as in *The Parable of the Talents* (a "talent" in this instance is said to be currency equivalent to about twenty years of wages for a labourer). The servant who looked after the talents he was given to manage by investing them and increasing their value, was given more by the returning master to manage. The servant who just hid his talent in the ground and did not improve its value had to give what he had to the one who had looked after well what he was given. In addition, he was called "lazy and slothful".

When you learn how to take responsibility for and care with what you have, improve what you have and respond to challenges, this can set the foundation for greater abundance and more opportunities for growth. I have found that when I am around people or situations that trigger a negative response in me, I need to refocus on the fact that I can control my response and I don't need to match the negativity of the person or situation. This mindset leads to the best outcome. For example, I can choose to focus on what I can learn instead, or I may need to choose my associations more carefully.

The following phrase came to me when I was seeking to transform my state of mind from a discouraged state to be encouraged again:

You can choose to wallow in self-pity,
or you can choose to work on bringing
your greatest dream to life.

There is always the power of choice available to you around how you'll respond to your circumstances as well as your attitude and mindset.

Exercise

Evaluate what you are choosing right now in your life. Is it helping you to move closer to your dreams or further away?

FLEXIBILITY

Stand your ground but be flexible to change.

Just as bamboo bends gently with the breeze, you should be flexible and open to adjusting your strategy when faced with significant resistance. Things will usually improve, but, if you don't see improvement over time, it may be best to reassess and consider changing your strategy. Eventually, the best course of action can be found if you keep in mind your desired goal or outcome while being flexible in your approach.

In a storm, bamboo and palm trees are very resilient, as they can bend and adjust with the winds. Similarly, in times of difficulty, I have found it helpful to set aside stubbornness and ask myself, *"Is there something new I can learn here? Can I approach this situation with greater flexibility?"*

For example, if a goal has not materialised within the timeframe I set in advance, instead of abandoning the goal, I will extend the deadline and ask myself, *"Is there anything I need to learn or do differently to achieve this goal?"*

If you've set a lofty goal and aren't sure how to achieve it, don't be quick to dismiss it. Instead, consider adjusting your level of belief, and focus on improving your skill set to make the goal feel more attainable. Remember, the greatest growth happens when we strive for something challenging yet meaningful—a goal that, if achieved, would be a dream come true.

Another opportunity for flexibility is when you have an argument with someone. Rather than insisting on them seeing things from your point of view, see if you can understand more where this person is coming from and their perspective. You may find that the argument dissolves or you can agree to disagree.

PATIENCE

If we believe our dreams are too far away or out of reach, complacency and a lack of motivation to pursue them may occur. This can be countered by visualising your dream every day, stating affirmations of what you're aiming for and making small wins, such as keeping the commitment to wake up at a certain time. I like to think about three of my best things of the day at the conclusion of each day, as it helps to set the foundation for more great things to be experienced.

Celebrate the small wins of the day, and you will be encouraged to achieve bigger and better things as time goes on.

Take it one day at a time. It's important to plan, but just as important to live in the present. It's great to review dreams and plans often, but remember to give your seeds of success the time to grow and have patience. Great accomplishments require a clear vision, a solid plan and patience to see them come true.

Have patience through the storms of life and for your most cherished dreams to come true.

Wanting quick results often leads to a decline or going backwards in achievements. For example, sometimes my students expect to master tai chi in a short period of time. However, it often takes years to fully learn the form and perform it with energy, grace and ease. True mastery is a journey that requires patience, dedication and consistent practice.

Maintain your hope and positive expectation. Keep working on your skill set. You can't hurry love—if you do, the love will lack the foundational strength that is necessary for its growth. Don't worry about what cannot be changed; focus on what can be changed for the better.

What do you do when you're waiting for your dreams to come true? You build up resources and refine skills. When there are enough resources, you can then arrive at your dream in a position of power rather than scarcity and worry.

Take steps each day towards your dream, not being disheartened at how long it's going to take, but with joy in your heart, grateful to be alive on this journey of life and with a great dream and vision to steer the way.

Exercise

For the next 30 days, say to yourself often, "*This dream of mine is coming true. I have the means and skills to make it a reality.*"

DECISION TIME

Have you made the decision to live according to your highest values and potential? If you have truly made that decision, you will not waver in your commitment to the outcome. Yes, life may occasionally swerve you off the path, but, if you are dedicated to following your dream, you will get back on track and take action steps to realise it.

Decide what you really want and go for it. For instance, if you want to buy a home, avoid viewing properties that are less than ideal or that compromise your vision. Instead, focus on finding ways to raise the necessary funds for your dream home. Will enhancing your skill set help you achieve this?

How do you generate a knowing that is unshakable, that will see you through all the ups and downs? The answer lies in all the times you keep your commitments to yourself and God, no matter how small they are—for example, as not buying unhealthy foods when you are at the shops, showing up at the time you agreed upon for an appointment or completing the schedule you set the night before for the current day. Over time, these small actions accumulate, much like repeatedly saving small amounts of money grows into something significant. Soon, you will begin to see evidence of your greatest dream coming true.

When faced with a big decision, ask yourself the question: *"Will this have the effect of raising or decreasing my energy levels? Is this in alignment with my highest life vision and goals?"*

To be objective with decision making, try this simple exercise. Grab a piece of paper and draw a line down the centre. On the left side, list all the positives involved if you went ahead with the decision; on the right side, list the negatives you can see or feel could occur if you decline the decision. See which column has the most entries. This can be an indication of the best path to take.

If no answer appears straight away, be content with not having it just yet. You might need to gain more wisdom to make an informed decision. There are many great resources that can assist you, such as books written by those who have excelled in the area you wish to pursue. Stay open to learning new approaches and acquiring knowledge to guide you. It is good to have an idea of where you want to be and work towards it but also give yourself the time to be sensitive to inner and higher wisdom about the best path to take.

Exercise

When you have a major decision to make, write on a piece of paper all the options available to you. You may also list the positive and negative aspects of each, as you begin to sense and feel how you are with each option before you one by one. Is there a sense of peace and opening of energy? Or do you feel a constriction or uneasiness of energy? Where you feel peace, joy or harmony, this can be an indication of the best path forward.

WHAT IS HOLDING YOU BACK?

What you thought was an immovable difficulty could be a stepping stone to advancement.

What has held you back until now? When we ask ourselves this important question, it helps us find the answer to what has been troubling the mind or delaying progress in dream achievement. You have a choice in life to either sink into the hopelessness of old patterns or make a change for the betterment of yourself and the world.

For example, if I chose not to learn about marketing, how would people ever discover my online merchandise store or course? I realised the importance of stepping out of my comfort zone, researching effective marketing strategies and creating a plan to put them into action.

If you can overcome what is holding you back—be it learned helplessness, non-striving or non-achieving—by releasing it bit by bit, just like clearing away clutter, you will begin to see a path forming, and you will know in your heart what the next step needs to be. You cannot expect different results by doing the same things. Determine what needs to be changed and take action.

It may be a lack of finances that is holding you back, but don't let that stop you. It is good to identify your ideal vehicle for wealth creation while waiting for your dream to come true, so that, when you have the funds for your dream, you will also have the know-how to manage it well. You will have practised and learned the path towards success.

Sometimes, people say that a lack of funds is holding them back; however, with so much information and valuable knowledge available online with the click of a search button, there is much you can learn on whatever topic you wish to succeed in. Once you have raised the required funds, you will be knowledgeable on how best to proceed. In other words, you would have prepared well for new opportunities that could arise.

Your vehicle for wealth creation should ideally be something that you have an interest in and that you don't mind spending time to research how to excel in, whether it be learning how to succeed in business, property or shares. Find an area you have an affinity or resonance with.

For instance, if your dream is to be a great share trader and you don't have the money to trade, you can take several steps to prepare while building up your savings. Start by reading books on share trading by those who are successful in the field, listening to their insights on social media and learning as much as possible. This way, when you do have the funds to trade, you will not be starting from scratch; you will have a head start with your new knowledge and will know how to take a trade if it meets your trading criteria.

ENVIRONMENT

There is great beauty in simplicity. I believe our environment can inspire feelings of wealth or the opposite. If you are not yet in a place that makes you feel rich, why not visualise this place so you can have some clarity about what you are aiming for? Or, even if for a brief time, why not visit the place you dream about? Ideas may flow into your consciousness about how to achieve your dream.

For example, why not sit in a high-class restaurant or café and just sip coffee or tea while feeling the wealth and riches all around? Or you may like to visit the mountains or the beach to experience the emotions and beauty of nature and abundance.

Always aim to keep your environments at home and at work organised and neat to help manage the flow of abundance. To implement this, I make it a habit to clean and organise my desk and surroundings at the end of each workday. This way, when I start the next day, I come to a tidy and orderly workspace, allowing me to begin my work with ease and focus.

There are professional organisers who can assist if you find the task of clearing out unnecessary items at home too daunting. My sister, who has experience with decluttering, has greatly assisted me with learning how to declutter effectively. It is great to have a person who can help you look at your belongings objectively and assess if an item is needed or just taking up space.

Curiosity and wonder for life are amazing qualities to have. It is important to allow time for these qualities to develop and not to let this be tainted by all that needs to be done or obtained. Visiting new places while on holiday can help bring about curiosity and wonder. This can help fuel new insights into and inspiration about how to make improvements in life.

Exercise

Assess if your environment is supportive of your dreams and goals. Does it inspire you?

If not, what would be an environment that could inspire you? Can you spend some time there? Where is a high-energy area where you can gain an inspiring vision for the future? How can you improve your environment so it acts as a springboard that will propel you to high achievement?

Look at your calendar and check when you have scheduled your next vacation. If not scheduled yet, consider when you can get away for a time to regenerate and develop the qualities of new wonder and curiosity about life.

MEDITATION AS A MIND RESET

Whenever you're worrying too much or caught in a spiral of anxiety, a ten to fifteen minute meditation reprieve can work absolute wonders. Meditation can greatly assist in clearing the mind and helping to generate the right mindset and energy for your next endeavour.

I utilise meditation as a way to refresh my mind after intensely focusing on my work. After spending forty minutes of focused time on my to-do list tasks, I may sit quietly for seven to ten minutes and just focus on the breath. This not only gives the mind a break but also helps to re-energise the body, mind and spirit.

There is a wealth of information available about different approaches to meditation. One method involves maintaining good posture and focusing on the breath to cultivate calmness and clarity. Another is to pose a question that's been on your mind and listening patiently for the answer to emerge.

OVERCOME NEGATIVITY BY FOCUSING ON THE POSITIVE

Do your best to avoid dwelling on your problems and difficulties, as this can lower the energy of those around you. Instead, focus on the positive. Remember that what you focus on has the power to grow and shape your reality.

For example, when stuck in traffic, rather than letting impatience take over, I focus on where I would like to be in my life. I consider how I am traveling towards my bigger goals in life and think of ways I can improve my methods for achieving my dreams. I find that classical music, playing softly in the background, enhances this reflective process. Music with lyrics can be distracting, which is why I prefer classical. To overcome negativity, move into a high-energy state, assisted by a new environment, improved posture and breathing, and connection to inner joy. I have found that practising qigong and tai chi helps to achieve this high-energy state, especially when practised out in nature.

Let go of a lack of self-worth. Just like wiping a dirty window clean, allow the light of what your highest dream would look like and feel like to move into your consciousness.

Then, ask yourself, *"What can I do today to start the process of moving towards this dream realisation?"*

Another useful way to shift your focus from being negative to positive is to ask yourself, *"What is the small piece of gold I can gain from my current circumstance or event?"* It might be gaining empathy, patience or a strengthening of character. Realising what the gold is from the situation can reduce the negative vibration from the memory or circumstance you are facing at present.

Keep improving: Overcoming self-sabotage

There is a risk that, if one becomes very successful, there may be the temptation to self-sabotage. It is important at times of great success to continue to be discerning, keep up the practices which have made you successful in the first place and maintain your gratitude and appreciation. Keep learning how you can improve what you do and keep improving your skill set. This will help you to prevent self-sabotage and complacency.

Exercise

Evaluate any challenging situation you are experiencing right now or could face in the future and ask, *"What could be the gold or positive aspect of this challenge? How can it help me improve or become more accomplished than I am now?"*

Write down your answer in your journal.

PERSISTENCE

*Know the outcome you desire. Keep moving
towards this—don't stop.*

How long can you sit patiently, waiting for the conditions around you to magically improve? Are you doing all you can to be the best in all areas of life, or, somewhere along the way, have you lost the passion and zest to make it happen?

When nothing seems to be working, I would like you to ask yourself this question, *"Have I tried? Have I really tried?"* Persistence, my friend, can help to overcome obstacles.

I have found that asking the right questions helps build personal responsibility and personal power. When I don't achieve my desired results quickly, it is a signal that I may need to improve my knowledge in that particular area or practise greater patience.

*Take it one step at a time, one day at a time.
One dream at a time.*

Never give up on becoming all you can become. When you near the end of your life, there are some questions you would like to be able to answer "Yes" to with great sincerity: *"Did I do everything within my power to become all that I could become? Did I do all that I could to make this world a better place, not just for this generation but for future generations? Did my life have meaning, and did I share that meaning with others?"*

Exercise

Evaluate an area of your life that is not going as smoothly as you hoped it would be. Have you tried everything within your abilities to succeed in this endeavour? Determine what qualities are needed in your case. Is it more persistence, patience or skill development?

Record in your journal the answers to the above questions and a new plan going forward. Affirm often, *"Somehow, some way, I can make it."* Begin to implement your new plan of action.

POWER QUESTIONS

Questions can assist greatly with directing the focus of the mind. Write down your answers to the following questions:

- *Do I want to be someone who achieves their dreams or not?*
- *Am I doing all I can to be my very best?*
- *Do I have a "whatever it takes" attitude?*
- *What is my highest truth?*
- *What is it I yearn to be?*
- *What are my gifts?*
- *How can I make something great out of the resources I have?*
- *How can I be an example to others?*
- *How much of my highest potential am I tapping into?*
- *Am I keeping a firm faith that my wishes and dreams will come true, or am I worried it is taking too long?*
- *How can I nourish these dreams into reality, not just for my own sake but for all the lives I can help transform?*

I have learned from great mentors that we spend most of our time on what we value the most. So, whenever I catch myself procrastinating or spending too much time relaxing (if this time has not been scheduled as relaxation time), I ask myself, *"How important are my dreams to me? Do I truly value this dream?"* This reflection prompts me to revisit my calendar and the goals I set for the day, and I get back to work.

At times, we may need to ask the hard questions of ourselves, if we're not already achieving our desired results. These questions include: *"If being rich is so important to me, why am I not spending my spare time studying and learning how to make money work hard for me, rather than me working hard for money?"* and, *"If reaching my ideal body shape is so important to me, why am I not waking up early, putting on my exercise clothes and working out?"*

The excuses—I mean, answers—to the above questions are the reasons you're not taking action on your dreams. Look at them squarely in the face. This is what has been holding you back.

Now, let it go—no more holding back. Step into the light of what you can be.

STEP BY STEP

Whenever you are feeling discouraged, say this to yourself over and over: *"Step by step I will get there, one day at a time. If I continue to take small steps towards my greatest dreams, one day, they will amount to something great. One day, this dream will come true."*

To me, happiness occurs in the journey, when I am just calmly making progress bit by bit each day. Of course, it is lovely when the goal or dream is realised, but, most of the time, it is the working on the dream or goal and the feeling of improving over time that brings greatest peace and joy.

When you feel discouraged, bring to mind the times in your life when you felt the most encouragement. There was once a time when you felt vibrant and strong, and you can feel this way again. You are still the same person. Remember these feelings and stand how you would stand if you felt this way.

You have what it takes to achieve your dreams, one step at a time. You wouldn't have the dream in the first place if there weren't a chance you could achieve it.

Take heart, take courage. You can do it!

Exercise

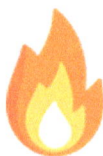

State the following with conviction and meaning:

> There is a little flame within that burns ever so softly and persistently.

> It says I can be something. I can make something of my life so wonderful that it will bring about my

greatest dreams, and, in the process, I can be an inspiration for others to achieve their dreams too.

All my life has been preparation for now. It's not too late to live my best life and become and achieve all I was created to become and achieve.

RECOGNISING INNER VALUE

Know your value and the value you bring to the world.

Failing to recognise your inner value often leads to unhealthy relationships and tolerating those that don't serve you. The opposite is also true: when you truly understand your value, you are able to recognise and appreciate others who share similar values, while also discerning those who fail to respect or acknowledge your worth.

When we do not fully accept our own inner value and recognise that we have something amazing to bring to the world, it can lead us to surround ourselves with people who drain our energy and bring us down. Sometimes, you need to take a hard look at the relationships in your life. Ask, *"Does this person uplift and inspire me when they are around? Or the opposite?"*

Form outstanding relationships with people who are supportive of dreams and are going somewhere in life—people who themselves are striving for greatness.

Decide which direction you would like to go in in life and make friendships and associations accordingly. If there is no-one in your inner circle of friends or family who inspires you, start to listen to inspiring mentors on YouTube and ask yourself, *"How can I find or be around people who are inspiring?"* Slowly but surely, over time, you can build a great network or team who will support and inspire you.

Knowing your value is also important in your career. Knowing my value as a writer has helped me create an online course, open a store with some of my best phrases on merchandise and write this book.

Exercise

Reflect on your inner value and how effectively you communicate and live out this value in your life.

DON'T SETTLE

Keep on keeping on.
Keep making progress.
You are closer than you think to
achieving your dream.

Don't settle in the valley if where you desire to be is on the mountaintop. Don't be influenced by quick fixes to achieve your dream.

A Japanese proverb states that, "Vision without action is a daydream. Action without vision is a nightmare." For example, settling for anyone who is not the person of your greatest dreams can only lead to bitter disappointment and regret.

In what ways have you made a compromise with your highest dreams, beliefs or values? Accepting what is merely okay doesn't leave much room for the wonderful and outstanding to appear. What is your highest and most wonderful vision of your life? Are you allowing this new way of life to be nourished into form by spending time on self-improvement, using your gifts and developing them? Or have you just accepted an "okay" way of life?

You can be outstanding. Believe you are worthy of great things happening in your life and that it is possible to bring to reality your highest visions. Do you need to lift your game by developing new routines and habits? We are what we continually do and envision. Do you want the next five years to be like the last five years? If the answer is no, then a different path is needed.

One practice that helps me avoid settling is committing to ongoing learning by reading books and attending seminars led by world-renowned experts in personal growth, business and finance. I've discovered that continual learning fosters consistent and steady personal and professional growth.

Study best practices and principles
and take action accordingly.
Know and connect to the highest truth in heart and
mind and, with inner joy, take that next step.

NO EXCUSES

Overcome all excuses and commit to the achievement of your dream.

Sometimes, we need to ask ourselves the tough questions if we are not where we had envisioned we'd be in life, or we need to remind ourselves of how fortunate we are. Have you forgotten how lucky you are? If you are healthy and have enough for food and essentials such as shelter, you really have no excuse for not striving to live your best life.

I state, "*No excuses,*" to myself if I require that extra motivation to commence a difficult task. I remind myself how lucky I am in many areas of life and then simply get to work.

The most important thing is to have a dream and believe you are worthy of this dream, then take the action steps to achieve it. If you find you are not taking the necessary actions, perhaps the dream is not compelling or strong enough.

State often, "*I am worthy of being rich in all areas of my life and of achieving my dream.*" You know what you can be and achieve by the vision you have when you close your eyes and ask yourself, "*Am I honouring the vision and potential I have been given by the way I am living my life?*" If the answer is no, you need to then ask, "*Why not? Is there anything in my life that requires clearing out or releasing? How can I best spend my time?*"

To help see the bigger picture in life, ask the question, "*How important will this issue be in five years?*" This usually places the issue faced into proper perspective.

AFFIRMATION OF SELF-WORTH

If every day you look in the mirror and say, *"I'm worthy of my dream. I have what it takes to be successful. I'm beautiful. I'm intelligent. I understand what I can do today to move closer to dream achievement,"* then, one day, as clear as the expansive blue sky, you will wake up and believe this to be true. Then, there will be no stopping you. You will take the necessary inspired actions towards your dream.

Our words are very powerful. I am often dismayed when I hear people say negative things about themselves, as they can often show up as our reality. If you ever look in the mirror and are not particularly happy with what you see, state the following, *"I am beautiful, and I have what it takes to be outstanding in all areas of my life."* Soon enough, you will begin to feel beautiful on the inside and outside. You may then be more likely to take the practical steps for better health and skin routines, such as exercising more or looking after your skin better by cleansing regularly and using a mud mask once a week.

It begins with self-belief.

Exercise

Practice the above affirmation as you look in the mirror each morning. Smile and state out loud, *"I am beautiful/handsome. I have what it takes to be successful in all areas of my life."*

HEALING OF LIFE

The boat has left the harbour.
Spirit has been rebuilt.
Slow and steady has won the race…

Healing and comfort can be obtained in each moment spent in reverence of the beauty of nature—the sunrise, the sunset—and in each moment you can let go of all fear and be totally present, listening to God's wisdom.

I believe that healing one's life begins in quietness, solitude and careful reflection. It's important to let go of the past and put it to rest while also holding on to the lessons that can guide you into the future. Meditation, writing down thoughts and dreams for the future, listening to inspiring faith-building messages, time in nature—these will all help with healing the mind, body and spirit. Remember the dream both when times are tough and when things are well. Always have something to strive towards.

It is through my practices that I strengthen my spirit and bring about the gentle healing of my life. I love to meditate and spend time in silence, as it is in these times that I have received answers to my prayers, such as the next step I need to take in my career for the greatest growth or a word of encouragement.

Exercise

Consider now if any area of your life is causing concern. Answer the following questions, in a quiet time of meditation:

- What inspired ideas could be a solution to this challenge?
- Is there a teacher who may already have a solution to this issue?
- What lessons can I learn from past challenging times?
- Am I ready to put this issue to rest so I can move forward to create the life of my greatest dreams?

INNER STRENGTH

Strength of spirit increases
each time you can say no to what is easy and
convenient but not right
and realign to higher truth and vision, taking
action in congruence.

Feel the strength within that you have what it takes to realise your dream—that no matter how long, how far, how many resources are required, or how much effort, you will be true to yourself and to your highest vision for life.

Don't settle in the valley of mediocrity and non-achievement through procrastination. Take a step each day, and you will move closer and closer to realising your highest vision and dream, inspiring others along the way.

Tap into that part of yourself that is strong and believes anything is possible. Discover the inner strength you have within. You do have what it takes to make a difference. Inner strength is essential to great wellbeing and success in life.

Times of solitude in meditation and gratitude can help to build inner strength.

Amid the ever-changing world, it is important to have the inner strength not just to get by but to rise to your highest potential and also to work on and express your inner gifts. Not everyone is going to believe in me or my dreams, but I must believe in myself and pursue them, despite any objections. My dreams for the future are worth it.

What dreams do you have that are worth fighting for, that you are going to believe are possible despite any objections? What is the dream you have deep within? To really go for your dreams with determination, persistence and action, you need inner strength. That imagined future full of possibilities can be yours if you keep on keeping on, take a step each day towards living that life and never give up.

Inner strength develops each time you keep the small and big promises you make to yourself. It means you need to follow through on plans rather than giving in to procrastination or laziness. Inner strength is the calm, peaceful reservoir within that can be summoned up in times of need to bring support and encouragement to make it through whatever challenges you may face.

> *Difficulties serve an important purpose; they make you stronger.*

In every setback or challenge I've faced—whether it's a lack of interest when I've posted some of my best work on social media or dealing with unhappy clients—I've learned to tap into my inner strength to stay positive. I understand that not everything will go as planned, but there's a higher purpose and mission for my life. I need to keep taking action to stay aligned with that purpose.

Each time I get back on my feet and keep striving to be my best, I build character and strength, so that, next time a challenge is faced, I have greater resources and know-how on how to navigate through or around the challenge.

CHAPTER 6

REVIEW AND INSPIRATION FOR THE JOURNEY

Successful living

*Know your dream and take a step each day
towards its achievement,
acknowledging inner and higher wisdom about the
best path forward.
With determination and strength of spirit,
never give up on your dream or give in to what is easy,
know that, somehow and some way,
against all odds,
you will become and achieve more than you ever
thought possible,
and, in the process, you will inspire others too.*

REFLECTION ON YOUR JOURNEY

When you see your dream beginning to be realised, take a moment to think back to how far you have come. How have you changed? Who have you become as a result of pursuing your great dreams that were once only a vision within? The difference you can now make in inspiring others to live their dreams makes the journey worthwhile.

Take the time now to reflect on your journey and how you have made changes in your life, such as taking the time to action the exercises in this book. Also reflect on the dreams you have achieved in your life and how far you have come in your journey.

Ten years ago, success to me meant having a tidy and decluttered home and sticking to my budget. Now, success means making a difference in the lives of others and inspiring them through my writing, whether that is through reminders of success in the form of phrases on merchandise or through books and workshops. I can see now that I have dreams today that I would not have conceived were even remotely possible in years gone by.

Our dreams and vision for the future can help us grow and achieve more than what we can imagine when daily action steps are taken towards their realisation.

Do you have something inspiring you are looking forward to? Take some time off for a holiday, away from your normal routine and in an inspiring environment. Time away can help bring you great insights on life improvement, goal setting and refining a great vision for the future. Always have something to look forward to. This can bring great inspiration and motivation to complete the mundane tasks in the meantime.

Exercise

What are you looking forward to or planning for? Take out your calendar and ask yourself:

- *What am I looking forward to?*
- *What am I planning for?*
- *Does this inspire me and help me to move closer to my dream achievement?*

THE PRESENT

Learn to live in the present,
not in the past, wishing,
"If only I had taken action on this matter,"
or in the future, wondering,
"What if this happens?"
What is important is what is here and now.
Just for this day, enjoy it for what it is,
for soon it will be washed away in the tide of time.

It is in the present moment that you'll find true magic and joy. It is also where you'll develop true awareness and focus. There are many who have had hopes and dreams for a better life but, through different circumstances, have not had the opportunity to live and experience their dearest dream and wish.

Every day, every moment in time, is a gift from God. We must use this time wisely and appreciate our blessings, doing our best to use our gifts and resources to the best of our ability, for we don't know what tomorrow will bring.

When moving forward to realise your greatest dream, don't forget to notice the beauty along the way—of nature, the flowers along the path, the breeze in your face, the taste of freshly brewed coffee, the sunsets and sunrises on the ocean.

To be fully present and appreciative of each day and each moment in time is to live, really live.

Don't think that only once you achieve all that is on your to-do list can you experience happiness and joy. Be happy and joyful now, happily and joyfully achieving your dream. How long are you going to wait to feel peaceful? With awareness and appreciation of each moment, you can feel this way now.

True power is in the present moment, directing energy and focus to the tasks at hand without distraction. Being truly present can help you accomplish great things.

Aside from meditation, the practices that most help me to be in the present moment are tai chi and qigong. These disciplines help clear the mind of distracting thoughts. Since I have practised the routines so often, they have become second nature. I don't need to think about what the next movement will be. I believe that true mastery is achieved when what you practise becomes an integral part of your daily life.

The power is in the present moment.
Savour this moment. Be in this moment,
fully present and aware.

LIFE'S GREATEST REWARDS AND LESSONS

Life does not reward the half-hearted, lukewarm dreamers and believers. Life's greatest rewards go to the ones who have unwavering faith and persistence and keep on keeping on until they see their great vision and dream realised. They then create a new one, always striving and believing they can improve and make a greater difference and impact, not just through their gifts and service to the world, but by their example.

Step up and become the highest version of who you
were created to be.

Life has a series of lessons. When we learn the lessons well and adjust our course to receive what we believe life is teaching us in the moment, life can flow with grace and ease. Great joy and peace arise when what we are doing is in alignment with what we are meant for.

As this book draws to a close, here are some final words of wisdom:

- Listen to what your inner wisdom and life is teaching you now and adjust your course if required.
- Live authentically and in the present moment.

- Utilise the gifts you have been given and contribute something wonderful to the world.
- Always have something to look forward to and have the courage to pursue your dreams.

Allow your light to shine. The world certainly needs it. There are many dark parts of our world that may need your assistance. Ask often:

- *Am I functioning at my best?*
- *Am I using my highest potential?*
- *How can I serve and be a blessing to a person in need?*

INSPIRATIONAL POEMS

The following are some inspirational poems and phrases that may assist you in your journey towards successful living and in achieving your dream.

Doorways

When one door closes,
another opens.
When one opportunity is lost,
another is on its way.
Be not concerned when all the doors seem to be closed,

*because it is when we are most challenged that the
spirit can rise up
in full glory and make its presence felt.
Step through that one door that is open to you now,
onto the path leading to your destiny.*

The heart's song

*Listen to the sound of your heart's true song.
Are you dancing in tune with this
or listening to the tune of outside influence?
The only way you can experience the true magic,
wonder and fulfillment of life
is to truly listen, acknowledge and take action in
alignment with what is truly in your heart.*

Beautiful day

*Notice the beauty that is in this day.
Dwell on all that is wonderful and things that you have,
not on perceived lack.
Believe all is well—great experiences and new
abundance are on their way.*

Give it your all

You never know what you are truly capable of if
you don't give it your all.
Give it your best, always, to honour the potential
given to you by God.

Inner truth

Shine brightly and acknowledge your inner truth.
You never know how many lives can be
transformed
by listening to inner wisdom and walking this path.

INSPIRATIONAL PHRASES

- Dig deep and remember the gift you bring to the world, your purpose and what brings joy to your heart.
- To thine own heart be true. Nourish greatest dreams into fruition by spending time each day on them.
- Step by step, you can make it. Focus on one thing at a time.
- You can be sad or get busy achieving your greatest dreams.
- Strive to be your best, no matter what the circumstance is.

- Each person is responsible for their own life. Life is what we make of it.

- Love gives meaning to life. It is the most exquisite feeling and state of being possible. Cherish this feeling and use its energy creatively for good.

- Great dreams come true if you believe.

- Be true to what is in your heart and actualise your highest vision for life.

- You haven't missed the boat. You just haven't tried.

- Don't compromise on your dreams—strive to reach them with everything you have.

- Great things are in store for those who are patient but work diligently towards their highest vision.

- Give from the heart with the intention of service.

- Step out in the pursuit of your dreams—they are beyond your comfort zone.

- Stay in gratitude for what you have in order for the good to continue.

- There are no limits to our potential except the ones believed or imagined.

- Trust all is well and will be well.

- You can do it. You can become and achieve all you have wished for and more, if you believe and take inspired action each day.

- Feel the strength within—you have what it takes to achieve this great dream. Believe and achieve.

- Fulfil your purpose and follow the calling of your heart.
- Value time and this moment—they are what life is made of.
- Keep up the momentum; your breakthrough is near.
- Practise excellence to experience excellence in life.

Thank you for taking the time to read this book. May you keep moving towards your dreams and living your best life. I wish you the best in your journey.

For more information and resources, such as courses and inspirational merchandise, please visit
www.wisdomandhealingqigong.com.au

ABOUT THE AUTHOR

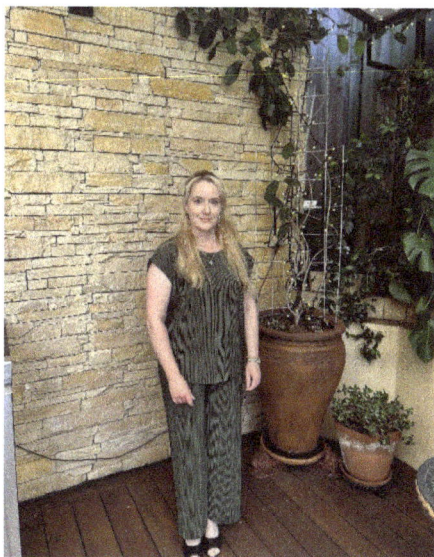

Catherine loves to spend time out in nature, where most of this book has been written. She has received training in science, acupressure, Reiki, life coaching, share trading, administration, tai chi and qigong, and has attended many personal growth workshops and seminars.

Today, Catherine is a writer of books, has an online store with her inspirational phrases on merchandise and is a course facilitator, tai chi instructor and share trader.

Her online course, **Healing of Life with Qigong and Inspirational Wisdom**, is available now.

Visit www.wisdomandhealingqigong.com.au for more information.

Online store: https://www.redbubble.com/people/GlimmeringDream/shop

ACKNOWLEDGEMENTS

I give thanks to God for helping me write this book and to my sisters—Susan, Anne and Alison—my mother, Coral, and my daughter, Shannara, for always believing in me.

Thank you to the teachers from all the courses I have attended and listened to online in personal growth and wealth creation, my personal trainer and instructors of karate and tai chi.

Thanks also to my editor and publisher.

www.ingramcontent.com/pod-product-compliance
Lightning Source LLC
Chambersburg PA
CBHW041718090426
42739CB00018B/3465